Lung Cancer

Editors

GANG CHENG
TIM AKHURST

PET CLINICS

www.pet.theclinics.com

Consulting Editor
ABASS ALAVI

January 2018 • Volume 13 • Number 1

ELSEVIER

1600 John F. Kennedy Boulevard • Suite 1800 • Philadelphia, Pennsylvania, 19103-2899

http://www.pet.theclinics.com

PET CLINICS Volume 13, Number 1
January 2018 ISSN 1556-8598, ISBN-13: 978-0-323-56647-6

Editor: John Vassallo (j.vassallo@elsevier.com)
Developmental Editor: Casey Potter

PET Clinics (ISSN 1556-8598) is published quarterly by Elsevier Inc., 360 Park Avenue South, New York, NY 10010-1710. Months of issue are January, April, July, and October. Periodicals postage paid at New York, NY, and additional mailing offices. Subscription prices per year are $232.00 (US individuals), $396.00 (US institutions), $100.00 (US students), $263.00 (Canadian individuals), $446.00 (Canadian institutions), $140.00 (Canadian students), $268.00 (foreign individuals), $446.00 (foreign institutions), and $140.00 (foreign students). To receive student and resident rate, orders must be accompanied by name of affiliated institution, date of term, and the signature of program/residency coordinator on institution letterhead. Orders will be billed at individual rate until proof of status is received. Foreign air speed delivery is included in all Clinics subscription prices. All prices are subject to change without notice. POSTMASTER: Send address changes to PET Clinics, Elsevier Health Sciences Division, Subscription Customer Service, 3251 Riverport Lane, Maryland Heights, MO 63043. **Customer Service: 1-800-654-2452 (U.S. and Canada); 314-447-8871 (outside U.S. and Canada). Fax: 314-447-8029. E-mail: journalscustomerservice-usa@elsevier.com (for print support); journalsonlinesupport-usa@elsevier.com (for online support).**

Reprints. For copies of 100 or more of articles in this publication, please contact the Commercial Reprints Department, Elsevier Inc., 360 Park Avenue South, New York, NY 10010-1710. Tel.: 212-633-3874; Fax: 212-633-3820; E-mail: reprints@elsevier.com.

PET Clinics is covered in MEDLINE/PubMed (Index Medicus).

Contributors

CONSULTING EDITOR

ABASS ALAVI, MD, MD (Hon), PhD (Hon), DSc (Hon)
Professor of Radiology and Neurology, Division of Nuclear Medicine, Department of Radiology, Hospital of the University of Pennsylvania, Perelman School of Medicine University of Pennsylvania, Philadelphia, Pennsylvania, USA

EDITORS

GANG CHENG, MD, PhD
Department of Radiology, Hospital of the University of Pennsylvania, Philadelphia, Pennsylvania, USA

TIM AKHURST, MBBS, FRACP
Associate Professor of Medicine, Nuclear Medicine Service, Cancer Imaging, Peter MacCallum Cancer Centre, The University of Melbourne, Melbourne, Victoria, Australia

AUTHORS

TIM AKHURST, MBBS, FRACP
Associate Professor of Medicine, Nuclear Medicine Service, Cancer Imaging, Peter MacCallum Cancer Centre, The University of Melbourne, Melbourne, Victoria, Australia

KHAMIS HASSAN BAKARI, MS
Department of Nuclear Medicine, Union Hospital, Tongji Medical College, Huazhong University of Science & Technology, Hubei Key Laboratory of Molecular Imaging, Wuhan, Hubei Province, China

KAI TOBIAS BLOCK, PhD
Associate Professor, Department of Radiology, Center for Advanced Imaging Innovation and Research, NYU Langone Medical Center, New York, New York, USA

FERNANDO E. BOADA, PhD
Director, Professor of Radiology, Psychiatry and Neurosurgery, Department of Radiology, Center for Advanced Imaging Innovation and Research, NYU Langone Medical Center, New York, New York, USA

HERSH CHANDARANA, MD
Associate Professor, Department of Radiology, Center for Advanced Imaging Innovation and Research, NYU Langone Medical Center, New York, New York, USA

GANG CHENG, MD, PhD
Department of Radiology, Hospital of the University of Pennsylvania, Philadelphia, Pennsylvania, USA

SARAH J. COUNTS, DO
Fellow, Cardiothoracic Surgery, Yale New
Haven Hospital, Yale School of Medicine,
New Haven, Connecticut, USA

SARAH EVERITT, PhD
Department of Radiation Oncology, Division of
Radiation Oncology and Cancer Imaging, Peter
MacCallum Cancer Centre, The Sir Peter
MacCallum Department of Oncology,
The University of Melbourne, Parkville,
Victoria, Australia

KATHRYN FOWLER, MD
Director of Abdominal and Pelvic MRI,
Assistant Professor, Department of Radiology,
Washington University in St. Louis, St Louis,
Missouri, USA

SAMUEL GALGANO, MD
Department of Radiology, The University of
Alabama at Birmingham, Birmingham,
Alabama, USA

LAEL GORE, CNMT, RT
Department of Radiology, The University of
Alabama at Birmingham, Birmingham,
Alabama, USA

HE HUANG, MD
Department of Nuclear Medicine, Luzhou
People's Hospital, Luzhou, Sichuan Province,
People's Republic of China

ANTHONY W. KIM, MD
Chief and Professor of Clinical Surgery,
Division of Thoracic Surgery, Keck School of
Medicine of University of Southern California,
Los Angeles, California, USA

THOMAS KOESTERS, PhD
Senior Research Scientist, Department of
Radiology, Center for Advanced Imaging
Innovation and Research, NYU Langone
Medical Center, New York, New York, USA

XIAOLI LAN, MD, PhD
Department of Nuclear Medicine, Union
Hospital, Tongji Medical College, Huazhong
University of Science and Technology, Hubei
Key Laboratory of Molecular Imaging, Wuhan,
Hubei Province, China

YIYAN LIU, MD, PhD
Nuclear Medicine Service, Department of
Radiology, Rutgers New Jersey Medical
School, University Hospital, Newark,
New Jersey, USA

MICHAEL MacMANUS, MD, FRANZCR
Department of Radiation Oncology, Division
of Radiation Oncology and Cancer Imaging,
Peter MacCallum Cancer Centre, The Sir Peter
MacCallum Department of Oncology,
The University of Melbourne, Parkville,
Victoria, Australia

JONATHAN McCONATHY, MD, PhD
Director of Molecular Imaging and
Therapeutics, Associate Professor,
Department of Radiology, The University of
Alabama at Birmingham, Birmingham,
Alabama, USA

MICHELLE McNAMARA, MD
Chief of GI Radiology, Associated Professor,
Department of Radiology, The University of
Alabama at Birmingham, Birmingham,
Alabama, USA

ALEXANDRE NIYONKURU, MS
Department of Nuclear Medicine, Union
Hospital, Tongji Medical College, Huazhong
University of Science and Technology, Hubei
Key Laboratory of Molecular Imaging, Wuhan,
Hubei Province, China

BENJAMIN SOLOMON, MBBS, PhD, FRACP
Medical Oncologist, Department of Medical
Oncology, Peter MacCallum Cancer Centre,
Melbourne, Victoria, Australia; Sir Peter
MacCallum Department of Oncology,
The University of Melbourne, Parkville,
Victoria, Australia

LAVINIA TAN, MBBS, FRACP
Medical Oncologist, Department of Medical
Oncology, Peter MacCallum Cancer Centre,
Melbourne, Victoria, Australia

JOHN V. THOMAS, MD
Chief of Body MRI, Associate Professor,
Department of Radiology, The University of
Alabama at Birmingham, Birmingham,
Alabama, USA

ZACHARY VIETS, MD
Department of Radiology, Washington
University in St. Louis, St Louis, Missouri, USA

Contents

and the development of effective targeted and immunotherapeutic agents have revolutionized the management of this malignancy. Although these therapies have resulted in improved outcomes for a subgroup of patients, their benefit may not necessarily be reflected by conventional response assessment criteria, because these therapeutic agents differ in their mechanism of action and response time compared with cytotoxic chemotherapy. Here the authors review available therapies in NSCLC and the utility of PET in therapeutic response assessment.

PET scanning plays key roles in planning the management of patients with lung cancer who are candidates for curative-intent treatment with radiotherapy and has contributed to improvements in survival. ^{18}F-fluorodeoxyglucose–PET is the most important modality for staging, patient selection, and radiotherapy target volume definition in patients with unresectable non–small-cell lung cancer. Developments include the availability of alternative tracers, such as ^{18}F-fluorothymidine, for imaging proliferation and a range of hypoxia imaging agents. The role of response-adapted therapy, based on interim PET scans performed during the treatment course, is being explored as a way of improving local disease control.

Non–small-cell lung cancer (NSCLC) is a leading cause of cancer-related death with a poor prognosis. Numerous factors contribute to treatment outcome. ^{18}F-fluorodeoxyglucose (FDG) uptake reflects tumor metabolic activity and is an important prognosticator in patients with NSCLC. Volume-based FDG-PET parameters reflect the metabolic status of a malignancy more accurately than maximum standardized uptake value and thus are better prognostic markers in lung cancer. FDG-avid tumor burden parameters may help clinicians to predict treatment outcomes before and during therapy so that treatment can be adjusted to achieve the best possible outcomes while avoiding side effects.

F18 Fluorodeoxyglucose (FDG) is a nonspecific PET tracer representing tumor energy metabolism, with common false-positive and false-negative findings in clinical practice. Non–small-cell lung cancer is highly heterogeneous histologically, biologically, and molecularly. Novel PET tracers designed to characterize a specific aspect of tumor biology or a pathway-specific molecular target have the potential to provide noninvasive key information in tumor heterogeneity for patient stratification and in the assessment of treatment response. Non-FDG PET tracers, including ^{68}Ga-somatostatin analogs, and some PET tracers targeting tumor proliferation, hypoxia, angiogenesis, and pathway-specific targets are briefly reviewed in this article.

There is an ongoing and successful effort in developing new radiopharmaceuticals that coupled with new developments in chemistry and instrumentation offers the potential of rapidly defining imaging biomarkers and theranostic paradigms. The overarching challenge remains in funding and approving such agents; the Food and Drug Administration in the United States is making efforts to improve the process, but the time to release PET agents from the regulator shackles is surely now, to bring to patients the excellence of preclinical work that has already been done.

Magnetic resonance (MR)/PET scanners provide an imaging platform that enables simultaneous acquisition of MR and PET data in perfect spatial and temporal registration. This feature allows improving image quality for the MR and PET images obtained during the course of an examination. In this work, the authors demonstrate the use of prospective MR-based motion tracking information for removing motion blur in MR/PET images of small pulmonary nodules. The theoretical basis for the algorithms is presented alongside clinical examples of its use.

Clinical PET/MR imaging is currently performed at a number of centers around the world as part of routine standard of care. This article focuses on issues and considerations for a clinical PET/MR imaging program, focusing on routine standard-of-care studies. Although local factors influence how clinical PET/MR imaging is implemented, the approaches and considerations described here intend to apply to most clinical programs. PET/MR imaging provides many more options than PET/computed tomography with diagnostic advantages for certain clinical applications but with added complexity. A recurring theme is matching the PET/MR imaging protocol to the clinical application to balance diagnostic accuracy with efficiency.

Modalities to detect and characterize lung cancer are generally divided into those that are invasive (endobronchial ultrasound, esophageal ultrasound, and electromagnetic navigational bronchoscopy) versus noninvasive (chest radiography, computed tomography, positron emission tomography, and magnetic resonance imaging). This article describes these modalities, the literature supporting their use, and delineates what tests to use to best evaluate the patient with lung cancer.

PET CLINICS

RELATED INTEREST

Radiologic Clinics,
November 2017 (Vol. 55, Issue 6)
Imaging and Cancer Screening
Dushyant V. Sahani, *Editor*
Available at: http://www.radiologic.theclinics.com/

THE CLINICS ARE AVAILABLE ONLINE!
Access your subscription at:
www.theclinics.com

PROGRAM OBJECTIVE

The goal of the *PET Clinics* is to keep practicing radiologists and radiology residents up to date with current clinical practice in positron emission tomography by providing timely articles reviewing the state of the art in patient care.

TARGET AUDIENCE

Practicing radiologists, radiology residents, and other health care professionals who provide patient care utilizing radiologic findings.

LEARNING OBJECTIVES

Upon completion of this activity, participants will be able to:
1. Review the use of PET/MRI in treatment planning for lung cancer.
2. Discuss the use of PET/CT imaging in diagnosing lung cancer.
3. Recognize prognostic factors for lung cancer.

ACCREDITATION

The Elsevier Office of Continuing Medical Education (EOCME) is accredited by the Accreditation Council for Continuing Medical Education (ACCME) to provide continuing medical education for physicians.

The EOCME designates this enduring material for a maximum of 15 *AMA PRA Category 1 Credit*(s)™. Physicians should claim only the credit commensurate with the extent of their participation in the activity.

All other health care professionals requesting continuing education credit for this enduring material will be issued a certificate of participation.

DISCLOSURE OF CONFLICTS OF INTEREST

The EOCME assesses conflict of interest with its instructors, faculty, planners, and other individuals who are in a position to control the content of CME activities. All relevant conflicts of interest that are identified are thoroughly vetted by EOCME for fair balance, scientific objectivity, and patient care recommendations. EOCME is committed to providing its learners with CME activities that promote improvements or quality in healthcare and not a specific proprietary business or a commercial interest.

The planning committee, staff, authors and editors listed below have identified no financial relationships or relationships to products or devices they or their spouse/life partner have with commercial interest related to the content of this CME activity:
Abass Alavi, MD, MD (Hon), PhD (Hon), DSc (Hon); Khamis Hassan Bakari, MS; Kai Tobias Block, PhD; Fernando E. Boada, PhD; Hersh Chandarana, MD; Gang Cheng, MD, PhD; Sarah J. Counts, DO; Sarah Everitt, PhD; Anjali Fortna; Kathryn Fowler, MD; Samuel Galgano, MD; Lael Gore, CNMT, RT; He Huang, MD; Thomas Koesters, PhD; Xiaoli Lan, MD, PhD; Yiyan Liu, MD, PhD; Leah Logan; Michael MacManus, MD, FRANZCR; Michelle McNamara, MD; Alexandre Niyonkuru, MS; Lavinia Tan, MBBS, FRACP; John V. Thomas, MD; John Vassallo; Rajakumar Venkatesan; Zachary Viets, MD.

The planning committee, staff, authors and editors listed below have identified financial relationships or relationships to products or devices they or their spouse/life partner have with commercial interest related to the content of this CME activity:
Tim Akhurst, MBBS, FRACP has stock ownership in PerkinElmer Inc.
Anthony W. Kim, MD is a consultant/advisor for Medtronic and F. Hoffmann-La Roche Ltd.
Jonathan McConathy, MD, PhD is a consultant/advisor for Avid Radiopharmaceuticals, a wholly owned subsidary of Eli Lilly and Company; Siemens Corporation; General Electric Company; and Blue Earth Diagnostics Limited, has stock ownership in Abbvie Inc., and his spouse/partner is a consultant/advisor for Abbvie Inc.
Benjamin Solomon, MBBS, PhD, FRACP is a consultant/advisor for Pfizer Inc; Novartis AG; AstraZeneca; Genentech, a Member of the Roche Group; Merck & Co., Inc; and Bristol-Myers Squibb Company.

UNAPPROVED/OFF-LABEL USE DISCLOSURE

The EOCME requires CME faculty to disclose to the participants:
1. When products or procedures being discussed are off-label, unlabelled, experimental, and/or investigational (not US Food and Drug Administration [FDA] approved); and
2. Any limitations on the information presented, such as data that are preliminary or that represent ongoing research, interim analyses, and/or unsupported opinions. Faculty may discuss information about pharmaceutical agents that is outside of FDA-approved labelling. This information is intended solely for CME and is not intended to promote off-label use of these medications. If you have any questions, contact the medical affairs department of the manufacturer for the most recent prescribing information.

TO ENROLL

To enroll in the *PET Clinics* Continuing Medical Education program, call customer service at 1-800-654-2452 or sign up online at http://www.theclinics.com/home/cme. The CME program is available to subscribers for an additional annual fee of USD $235.

METHOD OF PARTICIPATION

In order to claim credit, participants must complete the following:

1. Complete enrolment as indicated above.
2. Read the activity.
3. Complete the CME Test and Evaluation. Participants must achieve a score of 70% on the test. All CME Tests and Evaluations must be completed online.

CME INQUIRIES/SPECIAL NEEDS

For all CME inquiries or special needs, please contact elsevierCME@elsevier.com.

Preface
Lung Cancer

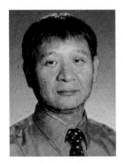 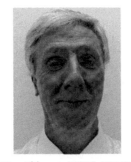

Gang Cheng, MD, PhD   Tim Akhurst, MBBS, FRACP

Editors

PET with fludeoxyglucose/computed tomography (FDG PET/CT) is widely used in pretreatment and posttreatment evaluations of various types of cancer, including non–small cell lung cancer. This issue of *PET Clinics* addresses the serious ongoing health problem of non–small cell lung cancer. The staging article summarizes the changes to TNM classification of lung cancer that have recently been announced. The lung neoplasms with low FDG avidity article expand on the problem posed by small nodules and those comprising predominantly ground glass opacities. It also introduces the concept that carcinoid tumors often have low FDG uptake. It is essential to recognize that the role of FDG imaging in these tumors is not tumor detection but assessment of the aggressiveness of the tumor, as the degree of FDG uptake in neuroendocrine tumors predicts growth rate. The prognosis article explores innovative assessment of the FDG signal in predicting outcomes of patients. It has long been known that the intensity of FDG uptake correlates with aggressiveness of a malignancy; the recent work examining the ACRIN data published this year is a dataset hard to ignore and shows that the metabolic tumor volume is prognostically important as would be expected. Intuitively, the greater the number of metabolically active cells, the greater the probability there will be cells harboring resistance to therapies. The Solomon article describes the impact of genomic analysis of lung cancers and illustrates why a targetable mutation is often better treated with a specific agent than a relatively nonspecific cell cycle agent, such as "conventional" chemotherapy. This is not to say that cell cycle approaches are not without validity, as is illustrated in the MacManus article on radiotherapy.

Non–small cell lung cancer has significant heterogeneity, which may exist within the same histological subtype, in different tumor masses of the same person or even within the same tumor mass. In addition to FDG, numerous new PET tracers are under development to evaluate other aspects of characteristic cancer biology in addition to glucose metabolism. 68Ga-somatostatin analogue PET imaging has significantly improved diagnosis of pulmonary carcinoid tumors versus other non-FDG–avid tumors and benign lesions. Most other new PET tracers targeting tumor proliferation, hypoxia, angiogenesis, or a specific signal pathway are under early development, with the potential to provide noninvasive and more specific information in tumor heterogeneity for better patient selection, treatment stratification, and therapeutic monitoring.

In terms of global health in decades ahead, the most challenging issue that faces us all is the rise of multidrug-resistant mycobacterium tuberculosis (TB). Increasing urbanization leads to greater frequency of person-to-person contact, especially as growing numbers of people utilize public transport. In addition, in today's global environment,

PET Clin 13 (2018) xi–xii
https://doi.org/10.1016/j.cpet.2017.10.001
1556-8598/18/© 2017 Published by Elsevier Inc.

international travel and relocation of refugees is becoming more common. The symptoms and signs of TB closely overlap with those of cancer; imaging findings on CT can mimic each other, and as pointed out in the article in this issue, FDG findings are also overlapping. Given the number of cases of people previously exposed to TB and the potential for reactivation, due to either the tumor or its treatment, increasing numbers of difficult cases will present. It seems both a challenge and an opportunity, a call to arms if you will, for governmental bodies to fund research into imaging TB itself. It would be a huge advance if lesions due to TB could be reliably distinguished from malignancy.

Gang Cheng, MD, PhD
Department of Radiology
Hospital of the University of Pennsylvania
3400 Spruce Street
Philadelphia, PA 19104, USA

Tim Akhurst, MBBS, FRACP
Nuclear Medicine Service, Cancer Imaging
Peter MacCallum Cancer Centre
305 Grattan Street
Melbourne 3000, Australia

E-mail addresses:
gang.cheng@uphs.upenn.edu (G. Cheng)
tim.akhurst@petermac.org (T. Akhurst)

Staging of Non–Small-Cell Lung Cancer

Tim Akhurst, MBBS, FRACP

KEYWORDS

- Non–small-cell lung cancer • TNM • Staging • FDG PET CT • EBUS

KEY POINTS

- The International Association for the Study of Lung Cancer has reevaluated the staging system for lung cancer, reviewing data from more than 100,000 patients with lung cancer.
- There are some changes in how T and M status are classified compared with the work completed in 2009.
- In addition, a major reworking of the classification of adenocarcinomas occurred in 2011.

TNM CLASSIFICATION

The International Association for the Study of Lung Cancer has reevaluated the staging system for lung cancer. Their analysis reviewed data derived from more than 100,000 patients with lung cancer. There are some changes in how T and M status are classified compared with the work completed in 2009. In addition, a major reworking of the classification of adenocarcinomas occurred in 2011. It is important that medical imaging reports reflect the new TNM (Tumour, Node, Metastasis) classifications. The UICC has already adopted the proposed changes. The American Joint Committee on Cancer has adopted the changes as well, but asked for a delay in implementation until January 2018 to allow software and databases to be updated and implement the new classifications.

T STATUS

The International Association for the Study of Lung Cancer has recognized the impact of screening and thinly sliced computed tomography (CT) scans on the types of lung cancer presenting for management. There has been an increasing number of early lung cancers detected. Careful evaluation of small lesions was undertaken to try to tease out differences in outcomes seen in T1 tumors (≤3 cm in diameter).

There is increasing recognition that fine cut CT characteristics of a lung nodule are important. The technology of CT scans outpaced reviews of the staging system such that lepidic tumor growth, now routinely detectable as a ground glass opacity (GGO) was previously classified as a malignancy despite no patients dying from such lesions. GGOs derive their name from the retention of the visualization of normal bronchovascular structures through the parenchymal opacity on CT imaging, and correspond with the presence of epithelial cells within alveolar walls. Where these lesions had been resected and where no solid component was present, essentially all patients survived. Lesions without an invasive component found at pathology that are less than 5 mm in size are now labeled atypical adenomatous hyperplasia. Lesions greater than 5 mm and less than 3 cm without an invasive component at pathology are now classified as carcinoma in situ, Tis, and are also nonlethal lesions.[1] There was considered insufficient evidence to conclude that lepidic lesions greater than 3 cm in diameter were benign and lesions of this size are called lepidic-predominant adenocarcinomas. It has been found that the areas appearing as solid on CT correspond to the invasive components found at pathology. The T1(mi) classification is new and reflects this. To classify GGOs accurately, 2 measurements need to be

Disclosures: None.

Nuclear Medicine Service, Cancer Imaging, Peter MacCallum Cancer Centre, University of Melbourne, 305 Grattan Street, Melbourne, Victoria 3000, Australia

E-mail address: tim.akhurst@petermac.org

PET Clin 13 (2018) 1–10

https://doi.org/10.1016/j.cpet.2017.09.004

made, first the diameter of the GGO and second the diameter of any solid component within the GGO, only the solid component should define the T1 subset[2] (**Fig. 1**).

As expected, there is a worse prognosis as tumors become larger. Each additional 1 cm in size has been proven to give a worse prognosis, up to lesions 5 cm in size. Lesions greater than 5 cm but less than 7 cm have a similar prognosis, and are grouped as T3. Lesions greater than 7 cm have a worse prognosis and are classified as T4.

The previous T4 descriptor of a tumor being less than 2 cm from the carina no longer was predictive of a worse outcome than T2 tumors and has, therefore, been removed as a descriptor.

Tumors that invade the diaphragm are now classified as T4 (this was not the case previously). The new classifications are as follows, with changes from the 7th edition italicized.

PRIMARY TUMOR

Tx = The primary tumor cannot be assessed, or tumor is proven by the presence of malignant cells in sputum or bronchial washings but cannot be visualized by imaging or bronchoscopy.

T0 = No objective evidence of a primary tumor.

Tis = Carcinoma in situ.

T1 is subject to subclassification, but is a parenchymal lesion (surrounded by lung or visceral pleura) equal to or less than 3 cm in maximal dimension, without bronchoscopic invasion of the main bronchus.

T1(mi) is a new classification that recognizes the excellent prognosis of minimally invasive adenocarcinomas, and is defined as a solitary adenocarcinoma less than or equal to 3 cm in diameter with a predominant lepidic pattern and less than or equal to 5 mm of invasion in any 1 focus.

T1a is an invasive tumor less than or equal to 1 cm in diameter or the uncommonly seen superficial spreading tumor of any length with invasion limited to the bronchial wall.

T1b is an invasive tumor greater than 1 cm in diameter but less than or equal to 2 cm in diameter.

T1c is an invasive tumor greater than 2 cm in diameter but less than or equal to 3 cm in diameter.

T2 is an invasive tumor greater than 3 cm in diameter but less than or equal to 5 cm in diameter or a tumor either (i) *involves the main bronchus but does not involve the carina* or (ii) invades the visceral pleura or (iii) *is associated with atelectasis or obstructive pneumonitis that extends to the hilum, involving part or all of the lung.*

T2a is a tumor greater than 3 cm in diameter but less than or equal to 4 cm in diameter.

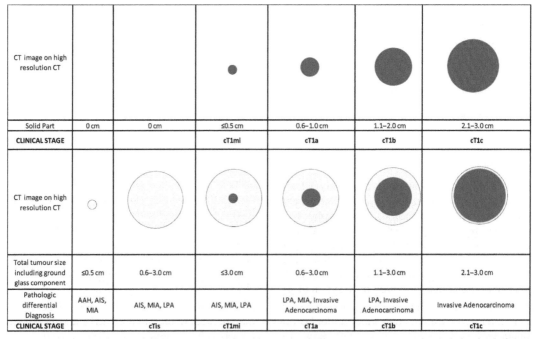

CT image on high resolution CT						
Solid Part	0 cm	0 cm	≤0.5 cm	0.6–1.0 cm	1.1–2.0 cm	2.1–3.0 cm
CLINICAL STAGE			cT1mi	cT1a	cT1b	cT1c
CT image on high resolution CT						
Total tumour size including ground glass component	≤0.5 cm	0.6–3.0 cm	≤3.0 cm	0.6–3.0 cm	1.1–3.0 cm	2.1–3.0 cm
Pathologic differential Diagnosis	AAH, AIS, MIA	AIS, MIA, LPA	AIS, MIA, LPA	LPA, MIA, Invasive Adenocarcinoma	LPA, Invasive Adenocarcinoma	Invasive Adenocarcinoma
CLINICAL STAGE		cTis	cT1mi	cT1a	cT1b	cT1c

Fig. 1. The solid component of lesions is in *blue*, the ground glass component is the lightly shaded area. Computed tomography scanning is part of clinical staging and that final staging involves pathologic evaluation, which can classify the pattern of a lesion's growth and the presence or absence of inflammatory or fibrotic change that can contribute to a nodule's size. AAH, atypical adenomatous hyperplasia; AIS, adenocarcinoma in situ; MIA, minimally invasive adenocarcinoma; LPA, lepidic-predominant adenocarcinoma.

T2b is a tumor greater than 4 cm in diameter but less than or equal to 5 cm in diameter.

T3 is a tumor *greater than 5 cm in diameter but less than or equal to 7 cm* in diameter or a tumor that either (i) *directly* invades any of the following: the chest wall (including parietal pleura and superior sulcus tumors), phrenic nerve,[a] parietal pericardium; or associated with a separate tumor nodule or multiple nodules in the same lobe as the primary.

T4 tumor is *more than 7 cm in diameter* or a tumor that invades any of the following structures: diaphragm, mediastinum, heart, great vessels, trachea, recurrent laryngeal nerve,[b] esophagus, vertebral body, or carina, or is associated with a separate tumor nodule or nodules in a different ipsilateral lobe to that of the primary tumor.

NODAL DISEASE

Nx: Regional lymph nodes cannot be assessed.

N0: No regional lymph node metastasis.

N1: Metastasis in ipsilateral peribronchial and/or ipsilateral hilar lymph nodes and intrapulmonary nodes, including involvement by direct extension.

N2: Metastasis in ipsilateral mediastinal and/or subcarinal lymph node(s).

N3: Metastasis in contralateral mediastinal, contralateral hilar, ipsilateral or contralateral scalene, or supraclavicular lymph node(s).

Distant Metastases

M0: No distant metastasis.

M1: Distant metastasis present.

M1a includes separate tumor nodule(s) in a contralateral lobe; a tumor with pleural or pericardial nodule(s) or malignant pleural or pericardial effusion. (It is recognized that the majority of pleural [or pericardial] effusions in patients with lung cancer are malignant but that cytologic specimens are often negative. A recommended pragmatic approach is that if the fluid is not bloody, not an exudate, that multiple cytologic examinations are negative, and the clinical impression is that the effusion is nonmalignant, that the effusion can be excluded as a staging descriptor.

M1b is a single extrathoracic metastasis. (This could be a single nonregional node.)

M1c is multiple extrathoracic metastases in 1 or several organs.

STAGING OF NEWLY DIAGNOSED NON–SMALL-CELL LUNG CANCER

To provide uniform datasets for analysis, trial entry and to attempt to give prognostic information, the TNM classifications for an individual patient are then combined together into an overall "stage." The new stage grouping are listed in **Table 1**.[4]

Table 1
TNM stage groupings

Stage	T Status	N Status	M Status
Occult cancer	Tx	N0	M0
Stage 0	Tis	N0	M0
Stage IA1[a]	T1a(mi)[a]	N0[a]	M0[a]
	T1a[a]	N0[a]	M0[a]
Stage IA2[a]	T1b[a]	N0[a]	M0[a]
Stage IA3[a]	T1c[a]	N0[a]	M0[a]
Stage IB	T2a	N0	M0
Stage IIA	T2b	N0	M0
Stage IIB	T1a-c[a]	N1[a]	M0[a]
	T2a[a]	N1[a]	M0[a]
	T2b	N1	M0
	T3	N0	M0
Stage IIIA	T1a-c[a]	N2[a]	M0[a]
	T2a-b	N2	M0
	T3	N1	M0
	T4	N0-1	M0
Stage IIIB	T1a-c[a]	N3[a]	M0[a]
	T2a-b	N3	M0
	T3[a]	N2[a]	M0[a]
	T4	N2	M0
Stage IIIC	T3[a]	N3[a]	M0[a]
	T4[a]	N3[a]	M0[a]
Stage IVA	Any T[a]	Any N	M1a
	Any T[a]	Any N[a]	M1b[a]
Stage IVB	Any T[a]	Any N[a]	M1c[a]

[a] Changes from the 7th edition.

Data from Goldstraw P, Chansky K, Crowley J, et al. The IASLC Lung Cancer Staging Project: proposals for revision of the TNM stage groupings in the forthcoming (eighth) edition of the TNM classification for lung cancer. J Thorac Oncol 2016;11(1):39–51.

[a]Phrenic nerve palsy is often quite apparent owing to elevation of the diaphragm, something most clearly appreciated on coronal images. Care needs to be taken to distinguish lung collapse leading to diaphragmatic elevation and phrenic nerve palsy per se.

[b]Recurrent laryngeal nerve palsies are characterized by 2 distinct and likely pathognomonic features, namely partial adduction (typically bowed centrally) of the affected side, seen on CT scanning, accompanied by asymmetric posterior cricoarytenoid muscle activity.[3] The posterior cricoarytenoid muscles abduct the cords and have to work harder on the contralateral side to maintain an adequate airway (Fig. 2). When a patient speaks during the uptake phase, activity can generalize along the nonparalyzed side. Of note, injection of the affected side is often undertaken to medialize the cord and increase voice production and improve cough; this outcome can induce a foreign body reaction that leads to ipsilateral laryngeal hypermetabolism. It is important to discuss with patients if such procedures have been done to reduce misinterpretation of the laryngeal findings.

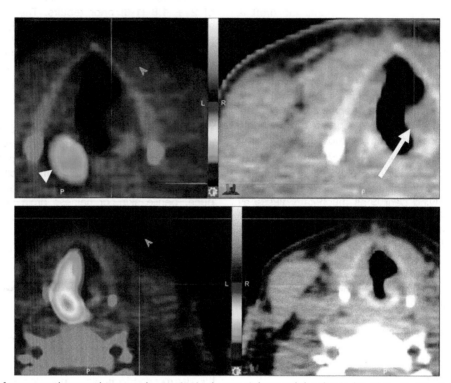

Fig. 2. Left recurrent laryngeal nerve palsy. Notice in the top right panel the classical "sail sign" of the left cord on CT with medial bowing of the posterior 1/3 of the cord (*white arrow*). This medialization leads to airway narrowing, and requires increased action of the opposite cord abductors to allow sufficient airflow. In this patient who did not speak during the uptake phase of FDG, the top left panel is a PET CT fusion image of the same study, the arrow head shows subtle asymmetrically increased uptake in the right posterior circoarytenoid muscle (whose action is to abduct the cord). This sign alone makes this patient T4. In the lower panels, a follow-up examination of the patient was performed, however this time, the patient spoke during the uptake phase. Notice how there is more generalized uptake through-out the larynx. A history needs be taken to rule out prior interventions, such as cord injection, that can themselves have FDG uptake related to the intervention. If that was to occur uptake would be ipsilateral to the paresis.

COMMENTS

1. It is likely that collaborative work like this will continue, and tumor parameters may move in or out of staging systems; academic centers interested in outcomes analysis should record raw data descriptors (such as tumor size in centimeters, number of nodes resected and number of nodes involved) in their databases rather than the TNM status alone. This would allow reanalysis of data using new classifications as they are adopted.

2. Recognizing that there can be additional peritumoral inflammatory changes, CT measurements of T size should include only the solid component of the tumor, the GGO component should be noted, but should not be considered part of the invasive component of the tumor for the purposes of TNM staging.

3. The daunting number of cases studied makes novel prognostic parameters unlikely to be included in staging systems, because the burden of proof required for acceptance is too high. Novel prognostic parameters derived from FDG PET CT datasets as described by Cheng and Huang (see Gang Cheng and He Huang's article, "Prognostic Value of ^{18}F-Fluorodeoxyglucose PET/ Computed Tomography in Non-Small-Cell Lung Cancer," in this issue), are more likely to be included in nomograms that aim to guide therapy rather than the TNM definitions per se. It is clear that, within a group of patients with lung cancer, subsets with specific actionable mutations will outlive others with no actionable mutations present.

THE ROLE OF PET WITH FLUDEOXYGLUCOSE F 18 COMPUTED TOMOGRAPHY SCANNING IN STAGING PATIENTS WITH LUNG CANCER

It has been shown that FDG PET CT scanning is better than CT scanning alone in determining nodal status and detecting occult metastatic disease than a contrast-enhanced CT scan[5] or a bone scan.[6] The timely detection of metastatic disease is by far and away the most important task when faced with a newly diagnosed lung cancer. Most patients with metastatic disease are not suitable for loco regional therapy with curative intent (**Fig. 3**).

It is now understood that osseous metastases establish themselves by coopting the environment established to foster hematopoiesis. Rapidly progressive osseous metastases occur in the red marrow space and do not alter cortical bone initially. Bone scans relying on phosphate metabolism are therefore insensitive in the detection of the marrow phase of osseous metastasis. FDG PET scans, by imaging the tumor itself rather than the body's response to the tumor, is more sensitive in the detection of osseous metastases than a conventional bone scan. When resectability of a primary lesion is in question, a contrast-enhanced CT scan should be performed to evaluate the relationship of the tumor to adjacent vessels and or bones. If a superior sulcus tumor is present and surgery is contemplated, an MR imaging examination is often requested to evaluate involvement of neural structures.

Nodal Disease

The incidence of nodal disease is related to the size of the primary tumor, and the pattern of nodal disease is relatively predictable. In terms of regional nodal drainage, it would be highly atypical for a left upper lobe tumor to spread to right-sided nodes without affecting left-sided nodes first, meaning that a solitary right hilar node is unlikely to be related to a left upper lobe lung cancer. Inflammatory processes arise typically owing to inhaled antigens and, because both lungs are exposed, usually give rise to symmetric nodal uptake. The pattern of symmetry is likely more relevant than the absolute uptake of FDG, because active granulomatous conditions can be very FDG avid. Another consideration is that nodes are likely to have metabolically similar cells within them to the primary lesion, and as a result a small intensely avid node is more likely to be malignant than a large node, that is, less avid than the primary tumor. These factors need to be borne in mind when interpreting FDG PET imaging findings (**Figs. 4** and **5**). Nodal disease can be biologically diverse; as an example compare **Figs. 6** and **7**.

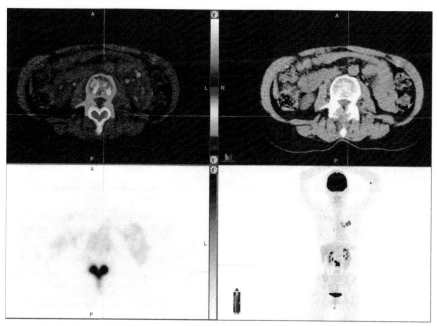

Fig. 3. Occult metastatic disease. This 58-year-old woman with a 30 pack-year history of smoking, having stopped 10 years ago presented with a hoarse voice, and a computed tomography (CT) scan of the chest was performed. This revealed a 33-mm left upper lobe partially necrotic mass with left hilar, aortopulmonary nodal involvement. An PET with fludeoxyglucose F 18 CT scan was performed to complete staging this revealed a previously unrecognized osteolytic L2 metastasis. The presence of a left vocal cord paresis renders her T4. She therefore has T4 N2 M1b, stage IVA disease.

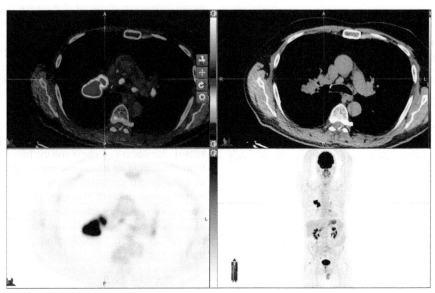

Fig. 4. This 60-year-old man presented with an ischemic arm, and computed tomography (CT) scanning revealed a 36-mm right perihilar mass with associated N1 adenopathy. A 17 × 11-mm precarinal node is mildly avid, as intense as the left hilar node, both a significantly less intense than the right hilar node. The PET stage of this tumor is N1 as the precarinal node would be expected significantly more intense if it were replaced with tumor. Activity in the base of the left ventricle is physiologic. To establish a diagnosis of malignancy, endobronchial ultrasound imaging will be required, if the precarinal nodes are confirmed to be benign this patient will have a T2a N1 M0 lung cancer.

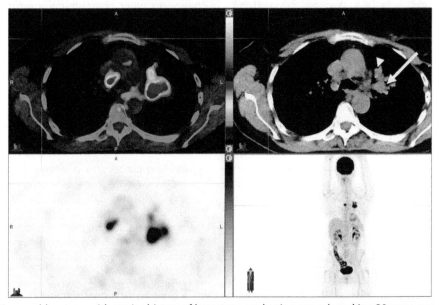

Fig. 5. A 66-year-old woman with a prior history of breast cancer, having ceased smoking 30 years ago, presented with headaches. A computed tomography scan of the chest was performed and showed an ill-defined left upper lobe tumor (*arrowhead*), a bulky left hilar node (*arrowed*), and a 17-mm right tracheobronchial angle node (N3). Endobronchial ultrasound imaging found a TTF-1–positive adenocarcinoma. Because surgery was unlikely to be successful, radical chemoradiotherapy was prescribed.

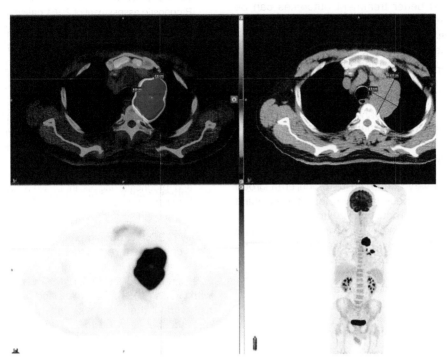

Fig. 6. N2 disease. Not all N2 disease is the same, as this case illustrates when the predominant node is not at all necrotic despite being 68 × 48 mm in size. It is likely the biology of this disease is very different from that seen in the patient in **Fig. 7**.

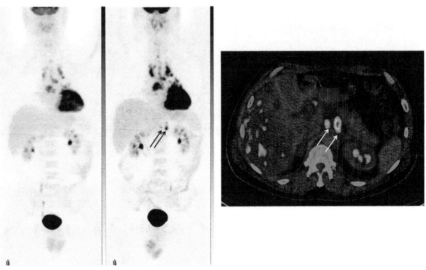

Fig. 7. A 43-year-old man with a 19 pack-year history of smoking presented with left sided pleuritic chest pain. A computed tomography (CT) scan was performed that revealed a left lower lobe mass, with ipsilateral, subcarinal, and contralateral nodes; these were confirmed by PET with fludeoxyglucose F 18 CT scan and subsequently mediastinoscopy found this to be a large cell carcinoma. He was deemed suitable for radical chemoradiation therapy and enrolled in a clinical trial that required reimaging with PET CT, which was performed 21 days after the initial PET CT. (*Right*) Baseline image. (*Middle*) New adenopathy can be seen in the upper abdomen (*arrows*), with interval increase in size and avidity of contralateral mediastinal nodes. The fused image on the *right* demonstrates the new nodal disease. This lead to a management change from chemoradiotherapy with curative intent to palliative chemotherapy.

Endoscopic Transbronchial Ultrasound Examination

Endoscopic transbronchial ultrasound examination is commonly used to stage the mediastinum and has to a large extent replaced cervical mediastinoscopy. Invasive cervical mediastinoscopy is less commonly performed because it disrupts the mediastinal soft tissues, making restaging the mediastinum difficult postinduction therapy,[7] and requires a general anesthetic. The use of endobronchial ultrasound imaging (EBUS) will vary according to which craft group the patient has been initially referred, because it is common for practitioners who can perform a procedure to do so. There are data to guide when to refer for EBUS. The literature comparing FDG PET with EBUS examination needs to be interpreted with care, owing to stage migration (that can occur at a rate that approximates 1% of patients per elapsed day) as was modeled by Everitt and colleagues[8] in a group of patients with predominantly stage III disease (see **Fig. 7**).

Gao and associates investigated the use of FDG PET imaging and EBUS scans in 329 patients presenting with T1 and T2 disease, of these 284 patients were classified as N0 by FDG PET. Surgical exploration revealed occult N2 disease in 7%. The negative predictive value of FDG PET was therefore 92.9%. As expected, T2 tumors had a higher incidence of occult N2 nodal disease (14 of 119; 11.8%) than T1 disease (6 of 165; 3.6%). The eighth edition T1 subclassifications further predicted incidence of N2 disease with 0 of 18 seen in T1a cases (0%), 2 of 78 in T1b cases (2.5%), and 4 of 68 in T1c cases (5.9%). They also found that the presence of a GGO was associated with a lower incidence of N2 nodal disease. N2 nodes occur in 15 of 119 patients (12.6%) with solid tumors, in 4 of 94 patients (4.3%) with semi-solid tumors, and 1 of 67 (patients 1.5%) with purely GGOs. Grouping patients with any ground glass component versus those with purely solid tumors lead to an incidence of N2 disease in 15 of 119 purely solid tumors (12.6%) versus 5 of 161 with GGOs (3.1%). They classified primary lesions as central if the lesion was within one-third of the distance between hilum and the lung periphery, or lateral if the lesion was in the outer two-thirds of the lung field. Applying this criteria seemed to be predictive, with 11 of 57 (patients 17.5%) with "central" tumors having occult N2 disease

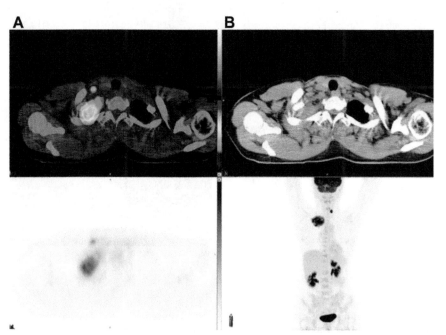

Fig. 8. A 48-year-old smoker with hemoptysis. PET with fludeoxyglucose F 18 revealed a 68-mm right pancoast tumor (T3) with an ipsilateral right supraclavicular node (N3), without hilar nor mediastinal nodal disease, and an incidental lesion in the left thyroid lobe. The left thyroid lesion would (*A*) rule out radical therapy and (*B*) is oncologically odd in terms of known patterns of spread, a biopsy was performed that revealed a papillary thyroid cancer. This rendered her M0. This allowed radical chemoradiotherapy to the right pancoast tumor and, upon recovery, a left hemithyroidectomy. The 35-month follow-up reveals no evidence of malignancy.

compared with 9 of 223 patients (4.4%) of with "peripheral" tumors. Combining tumor characteristics with tumor position was even more powerful, with solid central T2 tumors having a 33% risk of occult N2 disease, and peripheral T2 tumors with a ground glass component having a risk of 2%.[9] These data are consistent with other, previously published series.[10]

Comment

Careful evaluation of both FDG and CT data will allow identification of N0 cases in which an EBUS imaging is required. Peripheral T1 and T2 lung cancers with a GGO component staged as N0 on FDG, routine EBUS is unlikely to be beneficial. In contrast, central or T2 solid tumors should be referred for EBUS if the PET CT was N0 as the rate of mediastinal disease is more than 10%. Owing to the potential of stage migration, the workup and initiation of therapy needs to be expedited in patients with stage III disease.

The Importance of Biopsy

Aside from the important role tissue plays in selecting patients for specific targeted therapies, selected biopsy of oncologically odd lesions is important. An illustrative case is shown in **Fig. 8**, where a patient with a right pancoast tumor was staged with FDG PET scanning. There was no abnormal uptake in mediastinal nodes, a positive right supraclavicular node, making the patient T3N3Mx and potentially suitable for radical therapy. There was also a lesion adjacent to or in the left thyroid, that was also quite FDG avid, and if this was a metastasis, then curative intent radiotherapy would have been difficult to deliver. Although the supraclavicular nodal uptake is expected, the isolated skip lesion in the region of the thyroid is atypical for lung cancer. A biopsy of the left thyroid revealed papillary thyroid cancer, making the patient T3N3M0, stage IIIC (current classification; see **Table 1**). Radical chemoradiotherapy was administered, and after treatment a hemithyroidectomy was performed. The patient is recurrence free 33 months later. The teaching point of this case is that atypical lesions require further testing, particularly where management would be impacted.

SUMMARY

The staging of lung cancer serves 2 purposes. First, it attempts to classify patients into groups where particular treatments are appropriate. Second, staging has an important role in defining patient groups based on expected prognosis to allow design of clinical trials to test new therapies. The eighth edition of the International Association for the Study of Lung Cancer staging system deals with the issues raised by screening with fine cut CT scanning. Each phase of staging is a legitimate dataset on its own. The most accepted data are pathologic staging, but it must be recognized that pathologic staging is only as good as the imaging that guided the acquisition of tissue to arrive at the final stage. Finally, with the revolution of molecular testing leading to an increasing number of novel agents to treat systemic disease, the prognosis of individual patients will increasingly be determined by genetic susceptibility of the patient's specific cancer.

REFERENCES

1. Travis WD, Brambilla E, Noguchi M, et al. International Association for the Study of Lung Cancer/American Thoracic Society/European Respiratory Society International Multidisciplinary Classification of Lung Adenocarcinoma. J Thorac Oncol 2011; 6(2):244–85.
2. Travis WD, Asamura H, Bankier AA, et al. The IASLC lung cancer staging project: proposals for coding T categories for subsolid nodules and assessment of tumor size in part-solid tumors in the forthcoming eighth edition of the TNM classification of lung cancer. J Thorac Oncol 2016;11(8):1204–23.
3. Komissarova M, Wong KK, Piert M, et al. Spectrum of 18F-FDG PET/CT findings in oncology-related recurrent laryngeal nerve palsy. AJR Am J Roentgenol 2009;192(1):288–94.
4. Goldstraw P, Chansky K, Crowley J, et al. The IASLC lung cancer staging project: proposals for revision of the TNM stage groupings in the forthcoming (Eighth) edition of the TNM classification for lung cancer. J Thorac Oncol 2016;11(1):39–51.
5. Vansteenkiste JF. Lymph node staging in non-small-cell lung cancer with FDG-PET scan: a prospective study on 690 lymph node stations from 68 patients. J Clin Oncol 1998;16(6):2142.
6. Qu X, Huang X, Yan W, et al. A meta-analysis of (1)(8)FDG-PET-CT, (1)(8)FDG-PET, MRI and bone scintigraphy for diagnosis of bone metastases in patients with lung cancer. Eur J Radiol 2012;81(5): 1007–15.
7. De Leyn P, Stroobants S, De Wever W, et al. Prospective comparative study of integrated positron emission tomography-computed tomography scan compared with remediastinoscopy in the assessment of residual mediastinal lymph node disease after induction chemotherapy for mediastinoscopy-proven stage IIIA-N2 non-small-cell lung cancer: a Leuven Lung Cancer Group Study. J Clin Oncol 2006;24(21):3333–9.
8. Everitt S, Herschtal A, Callahan J, et al. High rates of tumor growth and disease progression detected on

serial pretreatment fluorodeoxyglucose-positron emission tomography/computed tomography scans in radical radiotherapy candidates with nonsmall cell lung cancer. Cancer 2010;116(21):5030–7.

9. Gao SJ, Kim AW, Puchalski JT, et al. Indications for invasive mediastinal staging in patients with early non-small cell lung cancer staged with PET-CT. Lung Cancer 2017;109:36–41.

10. Lee PC, Port JL, Korst RJ, et al. Risk factors for occult mediastinal metastases in clinical stage I non-small cell lung cancer. Ann Thorac Surg 2007; 84(1):177–81.

Lung Neoplasms with Low F18-Fluorodeoxyglucose Avidity

Yiyan Liu, MD, PhD

KEYWORDS

• Lung cancer • FDG PET/CT • FDG uptake • FDG avidity

KEY POINTS

- Although it is less common than false positive, false-negative F18-fluorodeoxyglucose (FDG) PET/computed tomography is also a dilemma because of low or absent FDG avidity of some lung cancers.
- Pathologic type and clinical stage of lung cancer are independent factors associated with FDG avidity.
- Adenocarcinoma in situ and carcinoid are the most common lung malignancies with low FDG avidity.
- Small lesion size is a significant factor associated with negative PET finding.
- Morphology of lung lesions on anatomic images is another factor affecting FDG avidity. Subsolid pulmonary nodules, ground-glass nodules, or ground-glass opacity may be sources of false-negative PET.

Lung cancers are traditionally divided into non–small cell lung carcinoma (NSCLC) and small cell carcinoma (small cell lung carcinoma [SCLC]), with the former accounting for 80% of the cases and the latter accounting for the remaining 10% to 15%.[1,2] SCLCs behave aggressively and are treated nonsurgically in most cases, whereas NSCLCs are often managed by a combination of surgery and adjuvant therapy. Recognition of the diversity of NSCLC has led to its subclassification, culminating in the World Health Organization's 2004 and 2015 classifications. Major types of NSCLC include adenocarcinoma, squamous cell carcinoma (SCC), and large cell carcinoma. SCLC is grouped with other tumors exhibiting neuroendocrine differentiation.[1,3] Less than 5% of lung cancers are lung carcinoid tumors, sometimes also referred to as lung neuroendocrine tumors. Most of these tumors grow slowly and rarely spread.

PET/computed tomography (PET/CT) with F18-fluorodeoxyglucose (FDG) is a powerful diagnostic tool in the evaluation of patients with indeterminate pulmonary lesions and differentiation between benign and malignant causes.[4] FDG is a glucose analogue that accumulates in malignant tumors exhibiting increased glucose metabolism. Biochemically, FDG is a nonphysiologic compound with a chemical structure very similar to that of naturally occurring glucose. Like glucose, FDG enters the cells through membrane glucose transporter proteins. Once FDG is phosphorylated into FDG-6-phosphate by hexokinase, it is trapped inside the cell and does not undergo further metabolism as glucose does. Malignant cells often demonstrate increased FDG accumulation because of increased membrane transporters,

Disclosure Statement: None.
Nuclear Medicine Service, Department of Radiology, New Jersey Medical School, Rutgers University, University Hospital, 150 Bergen Street, H141, Newark, NJ 07103, USA
E-mail address: liuyl@njms.rutgers.edu

increased intracellular hexokinase, and low glucose-6-phosphatase. A few additional factors may also contribute to increased FDG uptake in the tumor, for example, vascularity of the tissue, elevated mitotic rate of the cells, high number of tumoral cells per volume of tumor, and presence of inflammatory cells within the tumor.[5,6] FDG accumulates in the cell in proportion to its glucose metabolic activity and can be semiquantitatively measured by the standardized uptake value (SUV). However, the intensity of FDG uptake on PET/CT may be affected by many physiologic and technical factors, including the blood glucose level, the time interval between FDG injection and image acquisition, patients' body composition and habitus, reconstruction technique, selection of region of interest, size of lesion, use of contrast agents during CT-attenuation correction, and so forth.

The National Comprehensive Cancer Network's guidelines recommend the routine use of FDG PET/CT scanning for the diagnosis of NSCLC. FDG PET/CT is very useful to distinguish between benign and malignant causes. Although specificity and positive predictive value are suboptimal because FDG is nonspecific for malignant tumors, and benign neoplasms and inflammation/infection may all demonstrate increased uptake, sensitivity and negative predictive value are excellent for characterization of pulmonary lesions. A meta-analysis investigating the accuracy of FDG-PET in diagnosing malignant pulmonary lesions estimated the sensitivity and specificity to be 96.8% and 77.8%, respectively.[7] A separate meta-analysis found the sensitivity, specificity, and accuracy of FDG-PET in the diagnosis of lung lesions to be 96%, 80%, and 91%.[8] However, there are some limitations of the diagnostic value of FDG PET/CT in lung cancer.[9] Although it is less common than false positive, false-negative FDG PET/CT is also a dilemma because of the low or absent FDG avidity of some lung cancers. This review discusses lung neoplasms with low FDG avidity on PET/CT and major factors influencing FDG uptake in lung cancer.

PATHOLOGY AND CLINICAL STAGE

The pathologic type of lung cancer is an independent factor associated with FDG avidity. In general, SCC, adenosquamous carcinoma, large cell carcinoma, and small cell cancer all demonstrate high FDG uptake on PET, whereas other tumors, such as low-grade adenocarcinoma, adenocarcinoma in situ (previously known as bronchioloalveolar carcinoma), well-differentiated adenocarcinoma, and carcinoid, may have low or absent FDG uptake.

Grogan and colleagues[10] reported a secondary analysis of the American College of Surgeons Oncology Group Z4031 trial for evaluating the accuracy of FDG PET/CT to diagnose clinical stage I NSCLC. False-negative scans occurred in 101 of 682 patients, with adenocarcinoma being the most frequent (64%) followed by squamous cell (11%), carcinoma in situ (10%), and neuroendocrine (9%). Only 11% of false-negative scans occurred in lesions sized less than 1 cm. The data suggested that pathology and clinical stage might affect the accuracy of FDG PET/CT.

In another study with surgical pathology correlation by Iwano and colleagues,[11] preoperative FDG PET/CT was false negative in 40 of 187 solid malignant lung lesions. With comparison of the characteristics between PET-positive and PET-negative lesions, there was no significant difference between 2 groups in body weight, blood glucose level, and tumor location. However, there was a statistically significant difference between 2 groups in histopathological types, clinical stages, and lesion size. Thirty-six of 40 lesions with false-negative PET were stage I. Adenocarcinoma in situ and well-differentiated adenocarcinoma had a tendency for negative PET findings.

In a study by Cheran and colleagues,[12] most PET-negative lung cancers were classified as stage I. In 20 patients with biopsy-proven primary lung tumors and negative PET studies at the time of presentation, tumor histology included 7 adenocarcinomas, 6 adenocarcinomas in situ, 3 carcinoids, 2 SCCs, and 1 otherwise unspecified NSCLC and 1 sarcomatoid neoplasm. Except for one patient with adenocarcinoma in situ and multifocal stage IV disease, all other patients were either stage IA (n = 14, 70%) or stage IB (n = 5, 25%). Eighteen (90%) of the 20 patients underwent curative surgical resection. No patient was known to have tumor recurrence after resection, and 3 (17%) of the 18 patients were known to be living and free of disease 5 years after surgery. With correlation to clinical follow-up information, the investigators found that with the exception of adenocarcinoma in situ and carcinoid, newly diagnosed lung cancers with negative PET findings were usually early stage diseases and associated with a favorable prognosis.

Among lung malignancies with low FDG avidity, adenocarcinoma in situ and carcinoid are the most common (**Fig. 1** and **Fig. 2**). Higashi and colleagues[13] investigated the correlation between FDG uptake and the degree of cell differentiation in 29 patients with 30 adenocarcinomas of the lung, including 7 adenocarcinomas in situ, 9 well differentiated, 2 well-moderately differentiated, 11 moderately differentiated, and 1 poorly

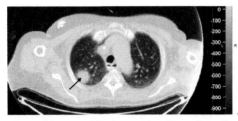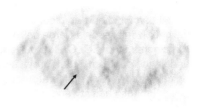

Fig. 1. A 72-year-old man with chest pain. CT workup showed a right lung lesion. FDG PET/CT demonstrated a 2.6 × 3.0-cm irregular mass with mild uptake (SUV 2.2) in the right upper lobe (*arrows*). There was no mediastinal lymphadenopathy or other abnormal finding. Surgical pathology from subsequent lobectomy suggested adenocarcinoma in situ.

differentiated. In 7 adenocarcinomas in situ, 4 lesions (57%) showed negative results on FDG PET, whereas in 23 other tumors, only 1 lesion (4%) had negative PET, which was a well-differentiated adenocarcinoma.

There are 2 separate clinical entities of adenocarcinoma in situ: focal and multifocal.[14] The focal variety has a better prognosis than other forms of lung cancer, whereas the multifocal form tends to behave aggressively, with a resultant poor prognosis.[15] Heyneman and colleagues[16] retrospectively reviewed 15 patients who had pathologically proven adenocarcinoma in situ and undergone FDG-PET imaging. Eight patients had focal adenocarcinoma in situ, and 7 patients had multifocal disease. Six of the 15 patients (40%) had negative PET scans; of these, 5 patients (83%) had the solitary form of disease. The sensitivity for focal tumors was only 38%, but the sensitivity for the multifocal form was 86%. The results suggested a high percentage of false-negative PET scans in the setting of focal adenocarcinoma in situ. However, in the presence of multifocal disease, FDG-PET seemed to be highly sensitive. The investigators assumed that multifocal adenocarcinoma in situ might have a different biological behavior than the focal form, despite a similar histopathology.

The mechanism of low FDG avidity of adenocarcinoma in situ is not well understood. Suzawa and colleagues[17] evaluated the major factors influencing FDG uptake in NSCLC by investigating the histologic difference in the expression of glucose transporters 1 and 3 (Glut-1 and Glut-3) and tumor size. Thirty-two tumors were analyzed, including 9 SCCs and 23 adenocarcinomas. The adenocarcinomas comprised 16 mixed subtypes and 7 localized adenocarcinomas in situ. The positive expressions of Glut-1 and Glut-3 were observed equally at high rates among SCC, adenocarcinoma mixed, and localized adenocarcinoma in situ, although the grade of expression of each Glut was the highest in SCC. For localized adenocarcinoma in situ, both FDG uptake and tumor size were significantly lower than those of lung cancers of the other two types. The results suggested that low FDG uptake in localized adenocarcinoma in situ was at least not primarily due to the difference in activities of Glut-1 and Glut-3.

Another pulmonary tumor that often has low FDG uptake is carcinoid, a neuroendocrine tumor. Pulmonary neuroendocrine tumors (pNETs) arise from bronchial mucosal cells known as enterochromaffin cells which are part of the diffuse neuroendocrine system. The pathologic spectrum of pNETs ranges from low- to intermediate-grade

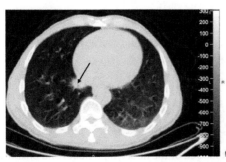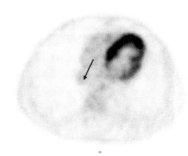

Fig. 2. A 60-year-old man with cough and infiltrate of the right lung on chest CT. FDG PET/CT showed a 2.8 × 2.2-cm subsolid pulmonary opacity with speculated borders and mild uptake (SUV 1.7) in the medial right lower lobe (*arrows*). CT-guided core biopsy was suggestive of a typical carcinoid.

neoplasms, such as bronchial carcinoids, including typical carcinoid and atypical carcinoid, to high-grade neoplasms, such as large cell neuro-endocrine carcinoma and SCLC. Typical carcinoids are indolent neoplasms that grow slowly and histologically show few proliferating tumor cells and minimal mitotic activity and with a good prognosis, whereas atypical carcinoids have a less indolent behavior with a certain propensity for metastatic spread.[18,19]

Although there were conflicting results of the detection rate of FDG PET/CT in lung carcinoids and some showed satisfactory results of FDG PET/CT,[20] most of published observations revealed a limited sensitivity of FDG PET/CT in lung carcinoids, especially typical carcinoids. In general, the sensitivity of FDG PET/CT seems to be overall higher in atypical carcinoids compared with typical carcinoids because of the more aggressive behavior and high proliferation rate of atypical carcinoids.[18]

Erasmus and colleagues[21] reported 6 of 7 pulmonary carcinoid tumors with negative PET findings. Jindal and colleagues[22] reported the imaging results of 20 patients with pulmonary carcinoids (13 typical and 7 atypical) on FDG PET/CT. Six of 13 typical carcinoids failed to reveal significant uptake on FDG PET/CT. All the atypical carcinoids revealed significant uptake on the FDG PET/CT that was higher than that in typical carcinoids.

Moore and colleagues[23] investigated FDG PET/CT findings in 29 patients with pathologic diagnoses of pulmonary carcinoids. Twenty-three were histopathologically typical, and the other 6 showed the atypical. The mean nodule size was 2.4±1.3 cm in the typical group versus 5.0±3.2 cm in the atypical group ($P = .065$). The mean SUV uptake in the typical carcinoid group was 2.7±1.6, and in the atypical group the SUV was 8.1±4.1 ($P<.01$).

Venkitaraman and colleagues[24] reported FDG PET/CT findings in 26 lung carcinoid tumors, including 21 typical carcinoids and 5 atypical carcinoids. The overall sensitivity, specificity, and accuracy of FDG PET/CT were 78.26%, 11.1%, and 59.37%, respectively. FDG PET/CT was true positive in all cases of atypical carcinoids and false negative in 8 cases of typical carcinoid (sensitivity for typical carcinoid 61.9% and for atypical carcinoid 100%, respectively).

Because carcinoids, especially typical carcinoids, usually show a lower metabolic activity compared with other lung carcinomas, Stefani suggested that an increased detection rate of FDG PET/CT in pulmonary carcinoids could be obtained by using a maximum SUV (SUV_{max}) cutoff lower than 1.5 and considering the normal lung, rather than the mediastinum, as background region for the visual assessment.[25]

SIZE OF LESION

It is well known that lesion size is a significant factor associated with negative PET findings (Fig. 3). Khalaf and colleagues[26] investigated the correlation between the size of pulmonary nodules and SUV on PET imaging in 173 patients. The SUV cutoff of 2.5 was used, and all patients had pathology biopsy. The results showed no or minimal value of FDG PET/CT in the evaluation of small pulmonary nodules less than 1.0 cm.

Li and colleagues[27] reported that the accuracy of FDG PET/CT improved with increasing size of

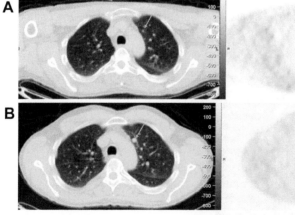

Fig. 3. A 56-year-old man with biopsy-confirmed metastatic SCC of the neck lymph nodes and unknown primary. The first PET/CT (A) demonstrated a non-FDG avid 0.5-cm pulmonary nodule in the left upper lobe (arrow). On repeated FDG PET/CT 5 months later (B), the nodule increased in size from 0.5 cm to 1.0 cm and had new FDG uptake (SUV 3.5). Surgical pathology confirmed a primary SCC.

pulmonary lesions: 64.2% in lesions less than 2.0 cm but 84.1% in lesions ranging from 3 to 5 cm. Lesions smaller than 2 cm may be falsely negative. Because SUV significantly correlated with tumor doubling time, those tumors with negative PET findings are likely to be slow growing and less avid.

Watanabe and colleagues[28] investigated the correlation between FDG PET/CT results and the clinicopathologic findings in 51 small lung cancers less than 3 cm in size. All of the 5 cases (4 adenocarcinomas and 1 small cell carcinoma) less than 1 cm in size were false negatives in FDG PET. In the 46 cases with lesions 1 to 3 cm in size, false-negative results were seen in 8 of 15 cases of well-differentiated adenocarcinoma (53%). Adenocarcinomas with a lesion size of 1 to 3 cm and false negatives on PET showed significantly less invasiveness than the true positives based on other clinical information, such as lymph node staging, vascular invasion, pleural involvement, and so forth.

The lack of visible uptake and/or low SUV in small lung lesions is secondary to so-called partial volume effect (PVE).[29] The PVE, also called limited resolution effect, is defined as a measurement error of the radiopharmaceutical concentration in regions with dimensions smaller than around 2 to 4 times the spatial resolution of the scanner.[30] When an object or structure being imaged only partially occupies the sensitive volume of the PET scanner, its signal amplitude becomes diluted with signals from surrounding structures, namely, the PVE.[29] In other words, PVE refers to that finite spatial resolution of the scanner produces an underestimation of radioactivity in small structures or lesions. In general, lesions smaller than twice the resolution of the imaging system may demonstrate the PVE. The PVE is a reason for a false-negative result of FDG-PET for small lesions.[31] In addition, PVE will also overestimate radioactivity adjacent to the hot area of a lesion and further decrease the radioactivity ratio of lesion to background.[32] PVE strongly depends on the size of the tumor; a smaller size of tumor is associated with a greater underestimation of the uptake value. Multiple models and methods are used or under investigation for correction of PVE. Several studies have shown that benign and malignant lesions, such as small tumors (<2 cm in diameter), were better distinguished with PVE correction than without.[33]

SUBSOLID NODULES

The morphology of lung lesions on anatomic images is another factor affecting FDG uptake. Subsolid pulmonary nodules, ground-glass nodule (GGN), or ground-glass opacity (GGO) may be sources of false-negative PET (see Fig. 2). Although most malignant lung lesions are solid in the anatomic images, such as CT, some may demonstrate subsolid nodules, GGN, or GGO. Subsolid nodules are now known to frequently represent the histologic spectrum of peripheral adenocarcinomas or well-differentiated adenocarcinoma, including adenocarcinoma in situ.[34]

In a prospective study by Nomori and colleagues,[35] FDG PET/CT scans were undertaken for 136 noncalcified nodules less than 3 cm in diameter. CT density histograms were made for each nodule to classify into solid and GGO. Eighty-one nodules were malignant and 55 were benign. All of the 20 nodules less than 1 cm in diameter (8 malignant and 12 benign) were negative on PET regardless of the histology. In the 116 nodules (101 solid and 15 GGO) sized 1 to 3 cm in diameter (73 malignant and 43 benign), 15 were negative on FDG PET. Among 15 GGO nodules, 10 were malignant and 5 were benign. All of the 10 malignant GGO nodules were histologically well-differentiated adenocarcinomas and 9 of them (90%) were false negative on PET. The sensitivity of FDG PET/CT for malignant nodules with GGO were only 10%.

Chun and colleagues[36] also reported the discouraging role of FDG PET/CT in the characterization of 68 GGNs with pathologic finding correlation. In partial solid nodules, the SUV_{max} was significantly higher in inflammation (2.00±1.18; range 0.48–5.60) than in malignancy (1.26±0.71; range 0.32–2.6). On the other hand, in pure GGNs, the SUV_{max} of malignancy (0.64±0.19; range 0.43–0.96) and inflammation (0.74±0.28; range 0.32–1.00) showed no difference.

Although there may be no or scant FDG uptake in malignant pure GGO nodules, a case report revealed that as the extent of solid component increases, PET had a tendency to show increasing FDG uptake.[37] Therefore, Godoy and colleagues[38] recommended a timely FDG PET/CT follow-up in GGOs with a mixed solid component, as they may represent a greater likelihood of being an invasive tumor.

LOW F18-FLUORODEOXYGLUCOSE AVIDITY AS A PROGNOSTIC IMPLICATION

Systematic reviews and meta-analyses revealed a negative correlation between the tumor SUV and aggressiveness and prognosis in patients with NSCLC.[39] The more metabolically active the tumor, the more aggressive it is and the worse the outcome.[40,41] Higashi and colleagues[41] reported a multicenter study to evaluate correlation between FDG uptake of primary NSCLC and intratumoral lymphatic vessel invasion and lymph node involvement in 132 patients. All patients underwent thoracotomy within 4 weeks of FDG PET/CT. Multivariate analysis was obtained, including age, sex, tumor size, histology, and FDG uptake. The results showed that only FDG uptake was a significant factor for intratumoral lymphatic vessel invasion and the FDG uptake and tumor size were significant factors for lymph node metastasis. In another study with 440 patients reported by Ishibashi and colleagues,[42] the tumor SUV_{max} was significantly lower in cases without intratumoral vessel invasion than those with positive intratumoral vessel invasion. The correlation between SUV_{max} and intratumoral vessel invasion was seen in both small and large lesions. Because intratumoral vessel invasion was closely related to lymph node metastasis, the intensity of FDG uptake on PET/CT can serve as an important pathologic marker of tumor invasion.

The prognostic value of SUV_{max} on FDG PET/CT for lung cancer has been widely reported in various staged diseases and kinds of populations.[43–47] A recent meta-analysis including 36 studies and total 5807 patients found that FDG PET/CT could be used for risk stratification in disease control and survival and could predict a high risk of recurrence or death in surgical patients with NSCLC.[39] Patients with high FDG uptake of the tumors may be considered at a high risk of treatment failure and may benefit from more aggressive treatment.

The biological basis for the prognostic value of FDG uptake in primary lung tumors is not fully understood; but upregulated glycolysis that results in increased FDG uptake has been associated with tumor growth, metastasis, and immune evasion.[48] Nair and colleagues[49] reported the identification of individual genes and gene expression signatures associated with prognostically relevant FDG uptake features. Fourteen quantitative PET imaging features describing FDG uptake were correlated with gene expression for single genes and coexpressed gene clusters (metagenes). Four of 8 single genes associated with FDG uptake were also associated with survival. The results were suggestive of additional gene expression involvement of FDG uptake except for changed glycolysis rate.

SUMMARY

Although FDG PET/CT demonstrates an accurate diagnostic role in lung cancer, false negatives may occur because of low or absent FDG avidity of some malignant lung neoplasms. Pathologic type and clinical stage are independent factors associated with FDG avidity. Among lung malignancies with low FDG avidity, adenocarcinoma in situ and carcinoid are the most common. Early stage disease often has low FDG uptake as well. Small lesion size is another significant factor associated with negative FDG-PET findings, which is due to PVE. The morphology of lung lesions on anatomic images may also affect FDG avidity. Subsolid pulmonary nodules, GGN, or GGO may be a source of a false-negative PET. Low FDG uptake of primary lung tumor is prognostic for less aggressiveness and favorable treatment outcomes.

REFERENCES

1. Zheng M. Classification and pathology of lung cancer. Surg Oncol Clin N Am 2016;25:447–68.
2. Travis WD, Asamura H, Bankier AA, et al. The IASLC lung cancer staging project: proposals for coding t categories for subsolid nodules and assessment of tumor size in part-solid tumors in the forthcoming eighth edition of the TNM classification of lung cancer. J Thorac Oncol 2016;11:1204–23.
3. Lewis DR, Check DP, Caporaso NE, et al. US lung cancer trends by histologic type. Cancer 2014; 120:2883–92.
4. Fletcher JW, Djulbegovic B, Soares HP, et al. Recommendations on the use of 18F-FDG PET in oncology. J Nucl Med 2008;49:480–508.
5. Kapoor V, McCook BM, Torok FS. An introduction to PET-CT imaging. Radiographics 2004;24:523–43.
6. Liu Y, Ghesani NV, Zuckier LS. Physiology and pathophysiology of incidental findings detected on FDG-PET scintigraphy. Semin Nucl Med 2010; 40:294–315.
7. Gould MK, Maclean CC, Kuschner WG, et al. Accuracy of positron emission tomography for diagnosis of pulmonary nodules and mass lesions: a meta-analysis. JAMA 2001;285:914–24.
8. Hellwig D, Ukena D, Paulsen F, et al. Meta-analysis of the efficacy of positron emission tomography with F-18-fluorodeoxyglucose in lung tumors. Basis for discussion of the German Consensus Conference on PET in Oncology 2000. Pneumologie 2001;55:367–77 [in German].
9. GUaron J, Dunphy M, Rimner A. Role of FDG-PET scans in staging, response assessment and follow-up care for non-small cell lung cancer. Front Oncol 2013;2:208.
10. Grogan EL, Deppen SA, Ballman KV, et al. Accuracy of fluorodeoxyglucose-positron emission tomography within the clinical practice of the American College of Surgeons Oncology Group Z4031 trial to diagnose clinical stage I non-small cell lung cancer. Ann Thorac Surg 2014;97:1142–8.

11. Iwano S, Ito S, Tsuchiya K, et al. What causes false-negative PET findings for solid-type lung cancer? Lung Cancer 2013;79:132–6.

12. Cheran SK, Nielsen ND, Patz EF Jr. False-negative findings for primary lung tumors on FDG positron emission tomography: staging and prognostic implications. AJR Am J Roentgenol 2004; 182:1129–32.

13. Higashi K, Ueda Y, Seki H, et al. Fluorine-18-FDG PET imaging is negative in bronchioloalveolar lung carcinoma. J Nucl Med 1998;39:1016–20.

14. Miller WT, Husted J, Freiman D, et al. Bronchioloalveolar carcinoma: two clinical entities with one pathologic diagnosis. AJR Am J Roentgenol 1978;130: 905–12.

15. Heikkila L, Mattila P, Harjula A, et al. Tumour growth rate and its relationship to prognosis in bronchioloalveolar and pulmonary adenocarcinoma. Ann Chir Gynaecol 1985;74:210–4.

16. Heyneman LE, Patz EF. PET imaging in patients with bronchioloalveolar cell carcinoma. Lung Cancer 2002;38:261–6.

17. Suzawa N, Ito M, Qiao S, et al. Assessment of factors influencing FDG uptake in non-small cell lung cancer on PET/CT by investigating histological differences in expression of glucose transporters 1 and 3 and tumour size. Lung Cancer 2011;72:191–8.

18. Lococo F, Cesario A, Paci M, et al. PET/CT assessment of neuroendocrine tumors of the lung with special emphasis on bronchial carcinoids. Tumour Biol 2014;35:8369–77.

19. Benson RE, Rosado-de-Christenson ML, Martinez-Jimenez S, et al. Spectrum of pulmonary neuroendocrine proliferations and neoplasms. Radiographics 2013;33:1631–49.

20. Alpay L, Lacin T, Kanbur S, et al. Are the 18F-FDG positron emission tomography/computed tomography findings in bronchopulmonary carcinoid tumors different than expected? Hell J Nucl Med 2013;16: 213–7.

21. Erasmus JJ, McAdams HP, Patz EF Jr, et al. Evaluation of primary pulmonary carcinoid tumors using FDG PET. AJR Am J Roentgenol 1998;170:1369–73.

22. Jindal T, Kumar A, Venkitaraman B, et al. Evaluation of the role of [18F]FDG-PET/CT and [68Ga] DOTATOC-PET/CT in differentiating typical and atypical pulmonary carcinoids. Cancer Imaging 2011;11:70–5.

23. Moore W, Freiberg E, Bishawi M, et al. FDG-PET imaging in patients with pulmonary carcinoid tumor. Clin Nucl Med 2013;38:501–5.

24. Venkitaraman B, Karunanithi S, Kumar A, et al. Role of 68Ga-DOTATOC PET/CT in initial evaluation of patients with suspected bronchopulmonary carcinoid. Eur J Nucl Med Mol Imaging 2014;41:856–64.

25. Stefani A, Franceschetto A, Nesci J, et al. Integrated FDG-PET/CT imaging is useful in the approach to carcinoid tumors of the lung. J Cardiothorac Surg 2013;8:223.

26. Khalaf M, Abdel-Nabi H, Baker J, et al. Relation between nodule size and 18F-FDG-PET SUV for malignant and benign pulmonary nodules. J Hematol Oncol 2008;1:13.

27. Li S, Zhao B, Wang X, et al. Overestimated value of (18)F-FDG PET/CT to diagnose pulmonary nodules: analysis of 298 patients. Clin Radiol 2014;69: e352–7.

28. Watanabe K, Nomori H, Ohtsuka T, et al. False negative cases of F-18 fluorodeoxyglucose-positron emission tomography (FDG-PET) imaging in small lung cancer less than 3 cm in size. Nihon Kokyuki Gakkai Zasshi 2004;42:787–93.

29. Keyes JW Jr. SUV: standard uptake or silly useless value? J Nucl Med 1995;36:1836–9.

30. Krempser AR, Ichinose RM, Miranda de Sa AM, et al. Recovery coefficients determination for partial volume effect correction in oncological PET/CT images considering the effect of activity outside the field of view. Ann Nucl Med 2013;27:924–30.

31. Salavati A, Borofsky S, Boon-Keng TK, et al. Application of partial volume effect correction and 4D PET in the quantification of FDG avid lung lesions. Mol Imaging Biol 2015;17:140–8.

32. Soret M, Bacharach SL, Buvat I. Partial-volume effect in PET tumor imaging. J Nucl Med 2007;48: 932–45.

33. Hickeson M, Yun M, Matthies A, et al. Use of a corrected standardized uptake value based on the lesion size on CT permits accurate characterization of lung nodules on FDG-PET. Eur J Nucl Med Mol Imaging 2002;29:1639–47.

34. Erasmus JJ, Macapinlac HA. Low-sensitivity FDG-PET studies: less common lung neoplasms. Semin Nucl Med 2012;42:255–60.

35. Nomori H, Watanabe K, Ohtsuka T, et al. Evaluation of F-18 fluorodeoxyglucose (FDG) PET scanning for pulmonary nodules less than 3 cm in diameter, with special reference to the CT images. Lung Cancer 2004;45:19–27.

36. Chun EJ, Lee HJ, Kang WJ, et al. Differentiation between malignancy and inflammation in pulmonary ground-glass nodules: the feasibility of integrated (18)F-FDG PET/CT. Lung Cancer 2009;65: 180–6.

37. Min JH, Lee HY, Lee KS, et al. Stepwise evolution from a focal pure pulmonary ground-glass opacity nodule into an invasive lung adenocarcinoma: an observation for more than 10 years. Lung Cancer 2010;69:123–6.

38. Godoy MC, Naidich DP. Subsolid pulmonary nodules and the spectrum of peripheral adenocarcinomas of the lung: recommended interim guidelines for assessment and management. Radiology 2009;253:606–22.

39. Liu J, Dong M, Sun X, et al. Prognostic value of 18F-FDG PET/CT in surgical non-small cell lung cancer: a meta-analysis. PLoS One 2016;11:e0146195.

40. Higashi K, Ueda Y, Arisaka Y, et al. 18F-FDG uptake as a biologic prognostic factor for recurrence in patients with surgically resected non-small cell lung cancer. J Nucl Med 2002;43:39–45.

41. Higashi K, Ito K, Hiramatsu Y, et al. 18F-FDG uptake by primary tumor as a predictor of intratumoral lymphatic vessel invasion and lymph node involvement in non-small cell lung cancer: analysis of a multicenter study. J Nucl Med 2005;46:267–73.

42. Ishibashi T, Kaji M, Kato T, et al. 18F-FDG uptake in primary lung cancer as a predictor of intratumoral vessel invasion. Ann Nucl Med 2011;25:547–53.

43. Imamura Y, Azuma K, Kurata S, et al. Prognostic value of SUVmax measurements obtained by FDG-PET in patients with non-small cell lung cancer receiving chemotherapy. Lung Cancer 2011;71:49–54.

44. Kim DH, Jung JH, Son SH, et al. Prognostic significance of intratumoral metabolic heterogeneity on 18F-FDG PET/CT in pathological N0 non-small cell lung cancer. Clin Nucl Med 2015;40:708–14.

45. Jeong YH, Lee CK, Jo K, et al. Correlation analysis and prognostic impact of (18) F-FDG PET and excision repair cross-complementation group 1 (ERCC-1) expression in non-small cell lung cancer. Nucl Med Mol Imaging 2015;49:108–14.

46. Kohutek ZA, Wu AJ, Zhang Z, et al. FDG-PET maximum standardized uptake value is prognostic for recurrence and survival after stereotactic body radiotherapy for non-small cell lung cancer. Lung Cancer 2015;89:115–20.

47. Yoo Ie R, Chung SK, Park HL, et al. Prognostic value of SUVmax and metabolic tumor volume on 18F-FDG PET/CT in early stage non-small cell lung cancer patients without LN metastasis. Biomed Mater Eng 2014;24:3091–103.

48. Koppenol WH, Bounds PL, Dang CV. Otto Warburg's contributions to current concepts of cancer metabolism. Nat Rev Cancer 2011;11:325–37.

49. Nair VS, Gevaert O, Davidzon G, et al. Prognostic PET 18F-FDG uptake imaging features are associated with major oncogenomic alterations in patients with resected non-small cell lung cancer. Cancer Res 2012;72:3725–34.

^{18}F-Fluoro-2-Deoxy-D-Glucose PET/Computed Tomography Evaluation of Lung Cancer in Populations with High Prevalence of Tuberculosis and Other Granulomatous Disease

Alexandre Niyonkuru, MS[a,b,1], Khamis Hassan Bakari, MS[a,b,1], Xiaoli Lan, MD, PhD[a,b,*]

KEYWORDS

- ^{18}F-fluoro-2-deoxy-D-glucose (^{18}F-FDG) • PET • Pulmonary tuberculosis • Lung cancer
- Standardized uptake value (SUV)

KEY POINTS

- ^{18}F-fluoro-2-deoxy-D-glucose (^{18}F-FDG) PET/computed tomography (CT) is widely used in the diagnosis of lung cancer and other malignancies. Increased ^{18}F-FDG activity on PET/CT imaging, as an indicator of tissue glycolytic activity, serves as a nonspecific tumor marker.
- Accumulation of activated macrophages and lymphocytes in active pulmonary tuberculosis also leads to increased uptake of ^{18}F-FDG in tuberculomas, which cannot be reliably differentiated from malignancy.
- The diagnosis of lung cancer using ^{18}F-FDG PET is compromised in tuberculosis endemic regions, because active tuberculosis granulomas cause significant false positive findings.
- Similar to tuberculosis, many other infections/inflammatory lesions, such as fungal infection, sarcoidosis, inflammatory pseudotumor, and so forth, may cause similar diagnostic dilemmas on ^{18}F-FDG PET imaging.
- In areas with a high incidence of tuberculosis, extra attention should be made to differentiate lung cancer from active pulmonary tuberculosis, so that unnecessary radical procedures can be avoided.

INTRODUCTION

Lung cancer is a leading cause of death by malignancy because of its high morbidity and mortality.[1]

Non–small cell lung cancer (NSCLC) accounts for more than 85% of all lung cancer cases.[2] ^{18}F-Fluoro-2-deoxy-D-glucose (^{18}F-FDG) PET/computed

---

Disclosure Statement: The authors declare that there was no conflict of interest.
[a] Department of Nuclear Medicine, Union Hospital, Tongji Medical College, Huazhong University of Science and Technology, Wuhan, Hubei Province 430022, China; [b] Hubei Key Laboratory of Molecular Imaging, Wuhan, Hubei Province 430022, China
[1] A. Niyonkuru and K.H. Bakari contributed equally to the article.
* Corresponding author. Department of Nuclear Medicine, Union Hospital, Tongji Medical College, Huazhong University of Science and Technology, No. 1277 Jiefang Avenue, Wuhan, Hubei Province 430022, China.
E-mail address: LXL730724@hotmail.com

PET Clin 13 (2018) 19–31
http://dx.doi.org/10.1016/j.cpet.2017.08.003
1556-8598/18/© 2017 Elsevier Inc. All rights reserved.

tomography (CT) has been well established as a crucial tool for detecting, identifying, and staging NSCLC, with obvious superiority compared with traditional anatomy imaging modalities.[2] A standardized uptake value (SUV) greater than 2.5 is often used as a cutoff value for differentiating lung malignancies from benign cases with ^{18}F-FDG PET/CT.[3,4] However, the specificity of ^{18}F-FDG PET/CT has been vigorously challenged. In clinical practice, it is not rare for benign lesions having an SUV higher than 2.5 and resulting in false positive diagnoses.[5]

Pulmonary tuberculosis (TB), caused by a Mycobacterium, is a common worldwide infection, especially in developing countries. It infects one-third of the world's population. Radiologically, it behaves like lung cancer[5-7] with variable manifestations. Such epidemic and radiographic features make pulmonary TB the leading cause of false positive PET/CT finding in lung cancer diagnoses in high prevalence areas, resulted in 57.1% to 92% of false positive diagnoses of primary lung cancer.[8-11] Because of activated immune cells, a TB site also presents an elevated level of glucose consumption,[12] difficult to differentiate from malignancies. Although efforts have been made, such as using delayed image acquisition,[9,13] this inherent shortcoming of ^{18}F-FDG has not been effectively solved.[10]

EPIDEMIOLOGY AND RISK FACTORS OF LUNG CANCER

Lung cancer is the leading cause of cancer deaths in both men and women in the United States. The incidence of lung cancer is higher in men than in women, but at present, the incidence is also increasing in women.[14]

Cigarette smoking is the primary risk factor for lung cancer.[15-17] Heavy smoking is associated with a 20- to 30-fold increase in lung cancer risk compared with nonsmokers. In general, 30% of lung cancers are squamous cell carcinoma, which is strongly associated with smoking. Squamous cell carcinomas, small cell lung carcinoma, large cell carcinoma, and to a lesser extent adenocarcinoma have an increased incidence with increased number of cigarettes smoked per day. Radon, a radioactive gas, is the second cause of lung cancer in the general population[18] and is the main cause of lung cancer in nonsmokers. Secondary smoking is the third leading cause of lung cancer.[19,20]

EPIDEMIOLOGY AND RISK FACTORS OF TUBERCULOSIS

TB is an airborne infectious disease caused by *Mycobacterium tuberculosis* (MTB) and is a major cause of morbidity and mortality, particularly in developing countries.[21-23] The global burden of TB is growing as reflected by increases in new cases and per capita incidence rates of 1.8% and 0.4% per year, respectively, between 1997 and 2000.[22] Worldwide there were 8.6 million new cases of active TB and 1.3 million deaths in 2012.[24] Most cases occur in Southeast Asia and Africa. The prevalence of TB in China accounts for 250,000 patients' annual deaths, the second highest worldwide.[25]

The risk for developing active TB is governed by exogenous and endogenous factors. Exogenous factors accentuate the progression from exposure to infection. Bacillary load in the sputum of the infected person, duration, and proximity to an infectious TB case are key factors. Endogenous factors, on the other hand, lead to the progression from infection to active TB disease.[26] Malnutrition, tobacco smoking, and indoor air pollution from solid fuel have been documented as the most important risk factors for TB worldwide, followed by HIV infection, diabetes, and excessive alcohol consumption.[27]

Extrapulmonary TB occurs in 10% to 42% of patients. The occurrence of the extrapulmonary disease depends on the age, presence or absence of underlying disease, ethnic background, immune status of the individual, and the strain or lineage of MTB.[26] The disease may occur in any part of the body and can mimic many clinical diseases, which potentially delays the diagnosis. HIV coinfection with TB presents major challenges to the diagnosis and treatment of TB.

PATHOPHYSIOLOGY OF TUBERCULOSIS IN RELATION TO ^{18}F-FLUORO-2-DEOXY-D-GLUCOSE UPTAKE

MTB is an aerobic, nonmotile, non-spore-forming rod that is highly resistant to drying, acid, and alcohol. It is transmitted from person to person via droplet nuclei containing the organism and is spread mainly by coughing. Invasion of the pulmonary alveoli with mycobacteria signals the start of TB infection, which later on invades and replicates within the alveolar macrophages.

Inhaled *mycobacteria* are phagocytized by alveolar macrophages, which interact with T lymphocytes, resulting in differentiation of macrophages into epithelioid histiocytes.[28] Epithelioid histiocytes and lymphocytes aggregate into small clusters, resulting in granulomas. In the granuloma, CD4 T lymphocytes (effector T cell) secrete cytokines, such as interferon-γ, which activate macrophages to destroy the bacteria with which they are infected. CD8 T lymphocytes (cytotoxic

T cell) can also directly kill infected cells.[29] Inflammatory cells such as neutrophils and activated macrophages at the site of inflammation tend to have more ^{18}F-FDG uptake.[30,31] Earlier studies have indicated that macrophages and lymphocytes in TB granulomas are responsible for high ^{18}F-FDG uptake on PET imaging.[31–34]

During the early stage of TB infection in the lungs, organisms commonly spread via lymphatic channels to regional hilar and mediastinal lymph nodes and via the bloodstream to more distant sites in the body. The main abnormalities are a progressive extension of inflammation and necrosis, frequently with development of communication with the airways and cavity formation. The endobronchial spread of necrotic material from a cavity may result in TB infection in the same or in other lobes. Hematogenous dissemination may result in miliary TB. The primary site of infection in the lungs is called the Ghon focus.[9] It either enlarges as the disease progresses or, much more commonly, undergoes healing. Healing may result in a visible scar that may be dense and contain foci of calcification.

THE ROLE OF ^{18}F-FLUORO-2-DEOXY-D-GLUCOSE PET/COMPUTED TOMOGRAPHY IN THE DIAGNOSIS OF LUNG CANCER

Early diagnosis and accurate staging are extremely important for the treatment of patients with lung cancer. CT, biopsy, and other examinations are routine methods in diagnosis and staging of lung cancer. However, increasing evidence suggested that incorporating ^{18}F-FDG PET imaging into the routine lung cancer diagnosis process could significantly improve the diagnosis and staging of lung cancer.[35] PET/CT imaging is used to differentiate between benign and malignant space-occupying lesions, which otherwise could be difficult to diagnose using conventional imaging modalities. The biggest challenge for PET/CT is in distinguishing benign from malignant solitary pulmonary nodule (SPN). Combining PET and CT is critical to overcome the false positive and false negative of the ^{18}F-FDG PET imaging.

In the diagnosis of pulmonary nodules, the lesion size, morphology, edge, density (eg, calcification, ground glass composition, air bronchial signs, and cavitation syndrome), growth rate, and the relationship between the nodule and the pleura are all important in the differentiation of benign and malignant lesions. The size of a nodule is the single most important risk factor for malignancy, regardless of its morphology: nodules with a size of 0.8 to 3 cm have an

18% risk of being lung cancer, and those that are more than 3 cm in size have a very high chance of being malignant. Irregular edge or spiculated margin, cavitary nodules or nodules containing small cystic spaces, and pleural tag are also suspicious for malignancy (**Fig. 1**). The most common CT manifestations of central-type lung cancer are the narrowing or obstruction of the bronchial lumen, hilar mass, and mass at the distal segmental or lobar atelectasis and consolidation on the side of the lesion. Moreover, lymphangitic carcinomatosis was typically seen in late-stage disease manifests as nodular interlobular septal thickening, which is usually asymmetric on imaging. Also, pleural metastases may appear as pleural nodules or pleural effusions.

Because most of the common primary lung cancers are ^{18}F-FDG-avid with the exception for a handful of lung cancers (such as well-differentiated adenocarcinoma, adenocarcinoma in situ [previously known as bronchoalveolar carcinoma], and some carcinoids), the metabolic activity of most lung cancers increased significantly. The evaluation of a lung lesion on ^{18}F-FDG PET includes visual analysis and semiquantitative analysis.[3,36–38]

Visual analysis is based on the level and morphology of radioactive uptake in the occupying lesions. The representative manifestation of PET imaging is a nodular or a clump of radioactive concentration that has a clear boundary (**Fig. 2**A–C). Cavities can be formed in the center of larger malignant tumors, which is characterized by a high concentration of radioactivity around the central radioactive defect. It is necessary to emphasize that many benign lesions also show increased metabolic activity. Therefore, a simple view of the metabolic degree of the lesions is not enough, and it is therefore very important that the morphology of the lesion with high radioactivity uptake on ^{18}F-FDG PET imaging should also be taken into consideration.

Semiquantitative analysis is performed according to the SUV of a lesion. The mean standard uptake value (SUV_{mean}) ≥ 2.5 is often used as a cutoff for judging pulmonary lesions as malignant with a sensitivity and specificity of 80% to 95% and 65% to 85%, respectively.[39–41] However, the ^{18}F-FDG uptake of pulmonary lesions, that is, the SUV, cannot be used as the sole diagnostic criterion. Being affected by many factors, it is imperative that one correctly understands its clinical value and its influencing factors. The SUV represents the activity of the radiotracer in a topographic region of the body image or volume of interest normalized to the weight of the patient

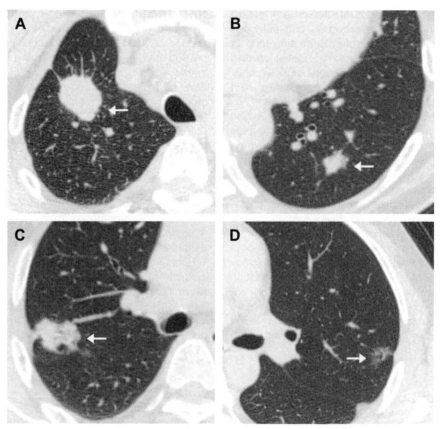

Fig. 1. Axial CT imaging. The arrow refers to the lesion, and all lesions were confirmed as lung cancer by pathologic diagnosis. (*A*) Irregular soft tissue mass with spiculated margin in the right lung. (*B*) A nodule with lobulated sign located in the lower lobe of left lung. (*C*) A nodule in the lower lobe of the right lung, accompanied by air bronchial sign, with adjacent pleural sag and pull. (*D*) A ground glass appearance nodule located in the superior lobe adjacent to the pleural of the left lung.

and to the quantity of radiotracer administrated, and it requires only a static scan with accurate instrument calibration, hence the formula:

$$SUV = \frac{Tissue\ activity\ (MBq/mL\ tissue)}{Injected\ dose\ (MBq)/body\ weight\ (g)}$$

which characterizes the relative concentration of the radiotracer in the lesion of interest. There are many factors affecting the value of SUV, such as acquisition interval after injection of ^{18}F-FDG, blood glucose and insulin levels, partial volume effect, the image acquisition mode (2-dimensional or 3-dimensional acquisition), image reconstruction model (the number of iterations), and so on.[4,9] Other clinical situations also need to be considered, including whether the patient has a history of smoking, age, gender, the shape of lung lesions, with or without extrapulmonary metastases. It is difficult to differentiate benign lung lesions with SUV close to 2.5 from lung cancer, especially for those nodular lesions that are less than 1.5 cm in size.

Numerous studies have reported on the use of ^{18}F-FDG PET imaging in the diagnosis of SPN and lung tumor.[42–44] Gould and colleagues[45] in their meta-analysis found that for pulmonary lesions, the overall sensitivity, specificity, positive predictive value (PPV) and negative predictive value (NPV) of ^{18}F-FDG PET imaging were approximately 96%, 78%, 91%, and 92%, respectively. Furthermore, a meta-analysis of 450 SPN cases showed that the sensitivity of ^{18}F-FDG PET in the diagnosis of lung cancer was 93.9%, specificity was 85.8%, and the median sensitivity and specificity were 98% and 83.3%, respectively.[46] In the literature, there are considerable differences in diagnostic sensitivity and specificity of lung cancer by ^{18}F-FDG PET/CT, depending on SUV cutoff selection, the size of a lesion, accompanying inflammatory granulomas, and other benign lesions. ^{18}F-FDG PET/CT has lower sensitivity for lesions less than 1 cm in size.

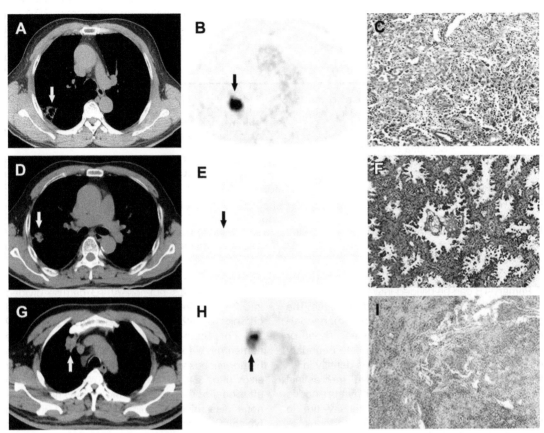

Fig. 2. (*A–C, D–F,* and *G–I*) Three different cases with true positive, false negative, and false positive images, respectively. (*A, D, G*) Axial CT images. (*B, E, H*) Axial ¹⁸F-FDG PET images. (*C, F, I*) Images of hematoxylin and eosin stain (original magnification: ×200, ×100, ×40). The arrow refers to the lesion. A high metabolic nodule (SUV$_{max}$ 11.7) located in the upper lobe of right lung was proved to be adenocarcinoma (*A–C*). Right lung upper lobe nodule with low uptake of ¹⁸F-FDG (SUV$_{max}$ 1.6) was confirmed as adenocarcinoma (*D–F*). High metabolic nodule locates in the right lung upper lobe (SUV$_{max}$ 7.9) was considered possibility a malignant tumor lesion, but the nodule was pathologically diagnosed as TB (*G–I*).

Like all imaging studies, ¹⁸F-FDG PET imaging has false negative (**Fig.** 2D–F) and false positive (see **Fig. 2**) diagnoses of lung cancer, and the latter could be as high as 20% to 25%. As an indicator of glucose metabolism, ¹⁸F-FDG can only be regarded as a broad-spectrum tumor imaging agent, and its uptake has significant overlap between tumors and nontumor tissues. It is known that activated mononuclear cells, leukocytes, and lymphocytes in granulomatous lesions have increased ¹⁸F-FDG uptake, mimicking lung malignancy. Common causes of false positive and false negative ¹⁸F-FDG PET/CT findings in the lungs are listed in **Table 1**.

THE ROLE OF ¹⁸F-FLUORO-2-DEOXY-ᴅ-GLUCOSE PET/COMPUTED TOMOGRAPHY IN THE DIAGNOSIS OF PULMONARY TUBERCULOSIS

About 60% of SPN are granulomas that can occur in any age group. Statistically, in young patients less than 35 years old with SPN, 90% of them were granulomas. Granulomas are mostly caused by TB, histoplasmosis, and coccidioidomycosis. In China, most of the granulomas in the lungs are TB. Round fibrous caseous necrosis with a diameter more than 2 cm are called tuberculoma, whereas diameter less than or equal to 2 cm are called tubercular nodules. The contents of the TB ball are mostly coagulated caseous necrosis, sometimes calcified, surrounded by fibrous coating with about 1 mm thickness.

The clinical classification of TB is important for differential diagnosis and treatment because clinical, pathologic, and imaging manifestations of TB are complicated, and each country has different classification methods. Herein, the authors briefly review the CT imaging of primary TB and hematogenous pulmonary TB. The possible difference in the CT characteristics between TB and peripheral lung cancer is listed in **Table 2**.

Table 1
Common causes of false positive and false negative ^{18}F-fluoro-2-deoxy-D-glucose PET/computed tomographic findings for suspected patients with lung cancer

	Classify	Diseases
False positive	Infectious diseases	Bacterial pneumonia, pulmonary abscess, pulmonary TB, fungal infection of lung (cryptococcosis, aspergillomycosis, coccidioidomycosis), bronchial fluke
	Granulomatous diseases	Active sarcoidosis, pneumoconiosis, Wegener disease
	Ischemia or necrosis	Pulmonary infarction
	Artifacts	Overcorrection caused by metallic implant materials or contrast agent; microembolism from precipitated tracer
False negative	Resolution-related factors	Small pulmonary nodules
	Few tumor cells	Mucinous carcinoma
	Low metabolism	Adenocarcinoma in situ, some carcinoids, or well-differentiated carcinoma

Primary TB can be divided into 2 types: primary complex and TB of intrathoracic lymph nodes. The characteristics of CT imaging for a primary complex show lobular alveolar nodules, sheet or patchy shadows with blurred lung field boundary (**Fig. 3**A), increased inhomogeneous density in lesions accompanied with hilar and mediastinal lymph nodes. The most common lymph nodes with increased inhomogeneous density are in homolateral hilar, superior vena cava, aortopulmonary fenestration, and subcarinal lymph nodes. CT imaging of TB intrathoracic lymph nodes shows single or multiple hilar and mediastinal lymph nodes with increased inhomogeneous density, which may be integrated into lumps. The density of these lesions in plain CT scan is inhomogeneous, with homogeneous enhancement in contrast-enhanced CT. If the density of the lymph nodes increases significantly and is associated with caseous necrosis in the center, these lesions may show a typical lymph node ring enhancement.

Hematogenous pulmonary TB can be divided into 2 types: acute miliary TB and subacute and chronic hematogenous disseminated pulmonary TB. For acute miliary TB, CT imaging shows numerous 1- to 2-mm miliary nodules distributed homogeneously in both lungs and with similar sizes (**Fig. 3**B). Some patients may have pleural effusion. For the subacute and chronic hematogenous disseminated pulmonary TB, CT imaging typically shows multiple pulmonary nodules with variable size and density, and some of them may have calcifications (**Fig. 3**C, D). These lesions tend to distribute differently in different parts of the lungs: lesions in the upper and middle lung fields are distributed more heterogeneously than those in the lower lung fields.

Although ^{18}F-FDG PET imaging of obsolete pulmonary TB is usually negative (**Fig. 4**A–C), active pulmonary TB often manifests high ^{18}F-FDG uptake (**Fig. 4**D–F). Active pulmonary TB mostly presents with high uptake of ^{18}F-FDG and irregular

Table 2
Differential diagnosis of tuberculomas and peripheral lung cancer on computed tomography

	Tuberculomas	Peripheral Lung Cancer
Primary sites	Superior lobe apicoposterior segment and lower lobe dorsal segment	Any part of the lungs
Size	2–3 cm mostly	More than 3 cm mostly
Morphology	Nonlobular or wavelike edge	Lobular
Margin	Smooth	Burr
Density	With calcification and cavities	Homogeneous
Satellite lesions	Commonly	Uncommon
Contrast CT scan	Nonenhancement or edge enhancement	Homogeneous enhancement or inhomogeneous enhancement

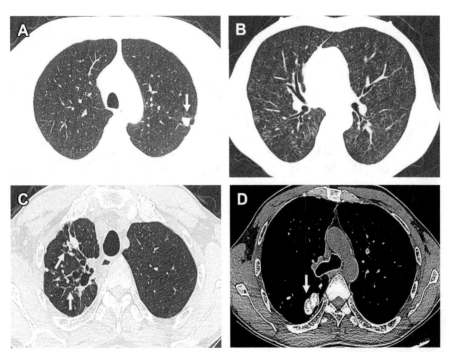

Fig. 3. Axial CT imaging, arrows showing lesions existence. (*A*) The tuberculoma can be seen in superior lobe of left lung. (*B*) Miliary opacities are present throughout both lungs. (*C*) Obsolete pulmonary TB showing pleural thickening, fiber lesions, and scarring. (*D*) A nodule with obvious calcification in inferior lobe of right lung.

distribution of the tracer. TB lymph node and pleural TB also show high uptake of ^{18}F-FDG (see **Fig. 4**). In addition, the SUV of active TB lesions continues to increase on delayed imaging, similar to that observed in lung cancer.[13]

Various reports have demonstrated that there is an association between bacterial burden and SUV in active TB granulomas.[47,48] Increased bacterial burden, especially during the early acute phase of infection, is responsible for increased ^{18}F-FDG uptake. Active TB granulomas between 3 and 6 weeks postinfection also have increased ^{18}F-FDG uptake, positively related to bacterial burden.[49]

PULMONARY TUBERCULOSIS: THE GREATER MIMICKER OF LUNG CANCER

Increased uptake of ^{18}F-FDG in tuberculomas can mimic lung cancer on PET/CT imaging. In areas with a high incidence of TB, active TB is a common pathologic process that interferes with the diagnosis of lung cancer on PET/CT[50] and leads to false positive results. SUV values are high in both TB and malignant lesions, with a significant overlap that limits the value of ^{18}F-FDG PET/CT.

Harkirat and colleagues[51] found that TB lesions have ^{18}F-FDG uptake patterns that are undifferentiated from that of lung cancer. They also reported

that active TB lesions may mimic other malignancies. Some TB lesions have SUV value up to 21.0 (range 2.2–21.0), which can easily mislead a physician to make a wrong diagnosis.[52] In a study by Goo and colleagues,[53] they observed 9 out of 10 patients with histopathologically proven pulmonary TB that showed ^{18}F-FDG uptake with a mean SUV_{max} value of 4.2 ± 2.2 on PET imaging.

Li and colleagues[8] in their study of 96 patients observed the sensitivity, specificity, accuracy, PPV, and NPV in the diagnosis of SPN were 86.7%, 72.2%, 81.3%, 83.9%, and 76.5%, respectively, for CT and 88.3%, 61.1%, 79.1%, 79.1%, and 75.9%, respectively, for PET. False positives of 57.1% (8/14) were due to TB on PET. The sensitivity, specificity, accuracy, PPV, and NPV in the diagnosis of SPN using PET/CT were 96.7%, 75.7%, 88.5%, 88.1%, and 94.4%, respectively. PET/CT accuracy was higher compared with that of either CT or PET alone ($P<.05$). They concluded that in an area with a high incidence of TB, PET alone has a high false positive rate. Moreover, combined PET and CT (PET/CT) can greatly improve the diagnostic accuracy in the differentiation of an SPN.

Sathekge and colleagues[9] evaluated 30 patients, who underwent dual time-point ^{18}F-FDG PET/CT imaging, followed by histologic examination of the SPN whereby the SUV_{max} with the

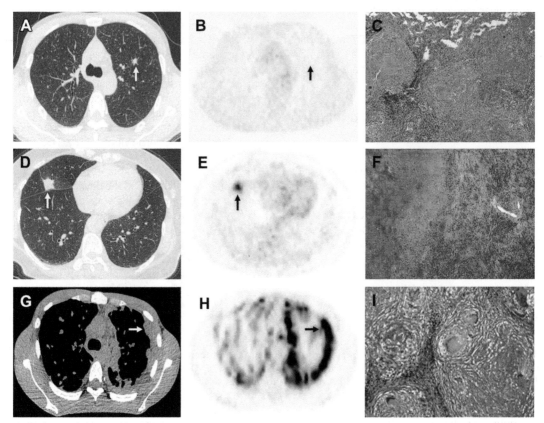

Fig. 4. (*A–C, D–F, G–I*) Three pathologic approved TB cases with different image features. (*A, D, G*) Axial CT images. (*B, E, H*) Axial ^{18}F-FDG PET images. (*C, F, I*) Images of hematoxylin and eosin stain (original magnification: ×40, ×40, ×200). The arrow refers to the lesion. (*A–C*) TB nodule in the upper lobe of left lung with low uptake of ^{18}F-FDG. (*D–F*) High metabolic TB nodule in the middle lobe of right lung. (*G–I*) Obvious high uptake through the pleura.

highest uptake in the lesion were calculated for 2 time-points (SUV1 and SUV2), and percentage change over time per lesion was calculated (% DSUV). After histologic confirmation, 14 were malignant lesions and 16 benign, of which 12 lesions were TB. The SUV1$_{max}$ for benign and malignant lesions were 11.02 (standard deviation [SD 6.6] vs 10.86 [SD 8.9]). Exclusion of tuberculomas from the analysis resulted in significant difference in mean SUV1$_{max}$ values between benign and malignant lesions (P = .0059). A sensitivity of 85.7% and a specificity of 25% were realized when using an SUV$_{max}$ cutoff value of 2.5, if all patients were included. However, a sensitivity of 85.7% and a specificity of 100% were obtained if TB patients were excluded from the analysis. There was no significant difference between mean %DSUV of benign lesions from mean %DSUV of malignant lesions (17.1% [SD 16.3%] vs 19.4% [SD 23.7%]), respectively. In addition, using a cutoff %DSUV greater than 10% suggestive of malignancy, a sensitivity and specificity of 85.7% and 50%, respectively, was realized. Excluding TB patients

from the analysis resulted in a sensitivity of 85.7% and a specificity of 75%. Therefore, they suggested that ^{18}F-FDG PET cannot differentiate malignancy from tuberculoma, and hence, is unreliable in the reduction of futile biopsy/thoracotomy in TB endemic areas.

Multiple studies have pointed out the importance of using dual time-point ^{18}F-FDG PET imaging in improving the accuracy of assessing SPN.[54–59] Accurate estimation of metabolic activity is only possible when SUV$_{max}$ is measured once ^{18}F-FDG uptake in tissues reaches its peak. However, ^{18}F-FDG uptake may continue to be elevated in some malignancies for several hours after tracer injection[60] despite the image acquisition time being approximately 60 minutes after tracer injection in most centers for the early imaging. Matthies and colleagues[54] in their study pointed out that ^{18}F-FDG PET imaging attained a sensitivity and specificity of 100% and 89%, respectively, when they assume an SUV increase of greater than 10% between the first and second scans as a cutoff point for malignancy. In this study, the single or first scan and second or delayed scan were initiated at a mean point of 69 minutes and 122 minutes, respectively, after tracer injection. Contrary to the above findings, Laffon and colleagues[61] established that neither an increase or a decrease in SUV can distinguish between benign and malignant nodules nor that dual time-point imaging (DTPI) was not suitable for lesions greater than 10 mm and with initial SUV_{max} greater than 2.5.

On the other hand, dual time-point ^{18}F-FDG PET/CT imaging is useful in differentiating active TB from inactive TB. A study by Kim and colleagues[13] focused on evaluating the role of dual time imaging with ^{18}F-FDG PET in the differentiation of active from inactive pulmonary tuberculoma in population of 25 patients with pulmonary tuberculoma. It found that active tuberculoma had higher values of SUV_{max} in both early and delayed phases (2.3 ± 0.75 and 2.48 ± 0.79, respectively) than those of inactive TB (0.79 ± 0.15 and 0.75 ± 0.13, respectively). Also, much difference of $\%\Delta SUV_{max}$ could be seen for the active and inactive TB (8.07 ± 7.77% and −3.83 ± 6.59%, respectively). Hence, the formula of $\%\Delta SUV_{max} = (SUV_{max}D - SUV_{max}E)/SUV_{max}E$ 100% ($SUV_{max}D$ = maximum SUV on delayed images, $SUV_{max}E$ = maximum SUV on early images). These results above suggest that the dual time-point ^{18}F-FDG PET imaging may be helpful for the differential diagnosis of active and inactive TB.

OTHER INFECTIOUS/INFLAMMATORY LESIONS MIMICKING MALIGNANCY

In addition to TB, there are multiple other active infectious and noninfectious inflammatory causes mimicking malignancy on ^{18}F-FDG PET/CT imaging. There are numerous reported false positive findings on ^{18}F-FDG PET imaging due to various granulomas other than TB. Previous study by Deppen and colleagues[62] observed that nearly half (46%) of the false positive ^{18}F-FDG PET scans in their population of 211 patients were due to granulomatous diseases. Furthermore, they also reported that 22 of 43 benign nodules (51%) were granulomas comprising 7 histoplasmoses, 2 blastomycoses, 1 sarcoidoses, 1 cryptococcosis, and 1 mycobacterium avium. The remaining 10 of 22 granulomas were indeterminate by initial pathologic staining.

Lung nodules that are fungal in origin may be metabolically active and appear similar to malignancy on both CT and PET (**Fig. 5A–C**), which is another common cause of false positive on ^{18}F-FDG PET scans. Accumulation of ^{18}F-FDG in

inflammatory cells is due to upregulation of cellular glucose metabolism secondary to respiratory burst.[63] Bryant and Cerfolio[64] found that 66% of ^{18}F-FDG PET false positive scans were due to fungal infections in the evaluation of pulmonary nodules. In fact, it has been recommended that ^{18}F-FDG PET could be used for the diagnosis and staging of invasive fungal infections.[65]

Sarcoidosis, a chronic noncaseating granulomatous disease predominantly in the lungs and lymph nodes, may involve any system. Sarcoidosis is often characterized by mediastinal bilateral symmetric enlargement of lymph nodes with high avidity of ^{18}F-FDG (**Fig. 5D–F**). It is a common cause of false positive findings involving multiple organs on ^{18}F-FDG PET imaging.[66] Multiple studies have observed that increased ^{18}F-FDG uptake in sarcoidosis makes it difficult in distinguishing between sarcoidosis and malignancy.[67–70] ^{18}F-FDG PET/CT is a useful and reliable imaging modality in the detection of pulmonary, extrapulmonary sarcoidosis (bone, liver, spleen, and retroperitoneal lymph nodes), monitoring, and treatment response and for the follow-up of patients with chronic persistent sarcoidosis.[71,72]

Inflammatory pseudotumor (IPT) is a rare but well-known benign process of unknown cause associated with both acute and chronic inflammation, with nonspecific radiologic features on either CT (which may appear as a lesion with low, equal, or high attenuation in relation to the surrounding tissue)[73,74] or on PET (high ^{18}F-FDG uptake) mimicking malignant processes in the lungs (see **Fig. 5**)[75,76] or other organs.[77,78] IPTs often have high level of ^{18}F-FDG uptake because of high density of inflammatory cells surrounded by fibrovascular stroma. The lungs are the most common localization of IPTs. Pulmonary IPT could be aggressive and exhibit malignant potential. With a high sensitivity (although low specificity) for IPT, ^{18}F-FDG PET/CT may be useful in monitoring therapeutic response of IPT lesions in postradiation, poststeroid therapy, and in those patients whose conditions precludes surgery.

Some studies suggested that the use of dual time-point ^{18}F-FDG PET/CT imaging is helpful in differentiation of granulomatous disease from malignancies. In a study conducted by Huang and colleagues,[79] involving 50 patients with SPNs in a region with endemic granulomatous disease, using dual time-point ^{18}F-FDG PET/CT imaging, the early imaging and delayed imaging were performed at 1 hour and 3 hours, respectively, postinjection of the radiotracer. On every pulmonary nodule, the SUV_{max} on early scans (SUV_{1h}) and delayed scans (SUV_{3h}) were calculated. Malignant

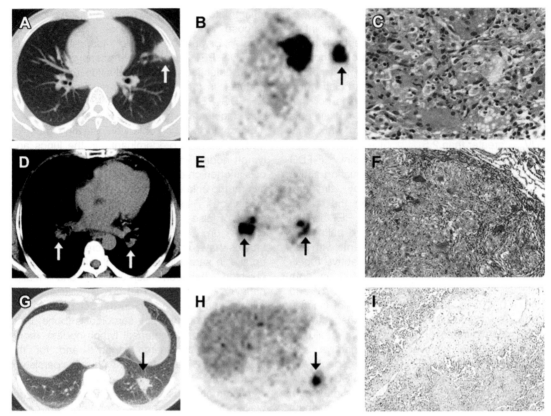

Fig. 5. (A–C, D–F, G–I) Three pathologic approved fungal, sarcoidosis, and IPT cases. (A, D, G) Axial CT images. (B, E, H) Axial 18F-FDG PET images. (C, F, I) Images of hematoxylin and eosin stain (original magnification: ×400, ×100, ×100). The arrow refers to the lesion. (A–C) A nodular mass adjacent to the pleura of the upper segment of left lung with high uptake of ^{18}F-FDG was confirmed as fungal. (D–F) Bilateral hilar enlargement lymph nodes with symmetric high uptake of ^{18}F-FDG were pathology proved to be sarcoidosis. (G–I) An IPT in the lower lobe of left lung shows obvious high uptake of ^{18}F-FDG.

and benign SPN were 37 and 13, respectively. Eight benign lesions out of 13 were found to be granulomatous diseases without specifying the histology of each granulomatous disease. The sensitivity, specificity, and accuracy of SUV_{1h} were 84%, 69%, and 80%, whereas for SUV_{3h} were 84%, 85%, and 84%. However, controversies exist. Chen and colleagues[80] reported in a retrospective study involving 149 patients in granulomas endemic regions using dual time-point ^{18}F-FDG PET/CT imaging to differentiate benign from malignant SPN. Their receiver operating characteristic analysis showed that the areas under curve (AUC) of early SUV_{max}, delayed SUV_{max}, retention index, single time-point imaging (STPI) PET/CT, and DTPI score were 0.73 ± 0.43, 0.74 ± 0.43, 0.61 ± 0.52, 0.77 ± 0.41, and 0.75 ± 0.45, respectively. The AUCs between early SUV_{max} and delayed SUV_{max}, and between STPI and DTPI PET/CT scores were not statistically significant (P = .48 and .36, respectively). The sensitivity, specificity, accuracy, PPV, and NPV

of the visual interpretation were 0.82, 0.65, 0.76, 0.83, and 0.62, for STPI PET/CT, and 0.79, 0.71, 0.77, 0.85, and 0.62 for DTPI PET/CT, respectively. No significant difference existed between STPI and DTPI PET/CT with visual interpretation. They concluded that, in granulomas endemic regions, DPTI PET/CT did not offer significant improvement over STPI PET/CT in differentiating benign from malignant SPNs in both quantitative analysis and visual interpretation.

SUMMARY

The uptake of ^{18}F-FDG serves as a nonspecific tumor imaging agent. It is known that mononuclear cells, leukocytes, and activated lymphocytes in granulomatous inflammatory lesions, in TB, and in many other infectious/inflammatory lesions, can increase ^{18}F-FDG uptake. In areas with a high incidence of TB, active TB often compromises the diagnosis of lung cancer on ^{18}F-FDG PET/CT and leads to false positive findings. In clinical practice,

PET/CT findings should be combined with patient's medical history, physical examination, and laboratory tests, to avoid misdiagnosis and unnecessary surgical procedures. Nevertheless, the final diagnosis may still require biopsy and pathologic confirmation.

REFERENCES

1. Torre LA, Bray F, Siegel RL, et al. Global cancer statistics. CA Cancer J Clin 2015;65:87–108.
2. Ettinger DS, Wood DE, Akerley W, et al. Non-small cell lung cancer, version 6.2015. J Natl Compr Canc Netw 2015;13:515–24.
3. Lowe VJ, Fletcher JW, Gobar L, et al. Prospective investigation of positron emission tomography in lung nodules. J Clin Oncol 1998;16:1075–84.
4. Hashimoto Y, Tsujikawa T, Kondo C, et al. Accuracy of PET for diagnosis of solid pulmonary lesions with 18F-FDG uptake below the standardized uptake value of 2.5. J Nucl Med 2006;47:426–31.
5. Shetty N, Noronha V, Joshi A, et al. Diagnostic and treatment dilemma of dual pathology of lung cancer and disseminated tuberculosis. J Clin Oncol 2014;32:e7–9.
6. D'souza MM, Mondal A, Sharma R, et al. Tuberculosis the great mimicker: 18F-fludeoxyglucose positron emission tomography/computed tomography in a case of atypical spinal tuberculosis. Indian J Nucl Med 2014;29:99–101.
7. Prapruttam D, Hedgire SS, Mani SE, et al. Tuberculosis: the great mimicker. Semin Ultrasound CT MR 2014;35:195–214.
8. Li Y, Su M, Li F, et al. The value of 18F-FDG-PET/CT in the differential diagnosis of solitary pulmonary nodules in areas with a high incidence of tuberculosis. Ann Nucl Med 2011;25:804–11.
9. Sathekge MM, Maes A, Pottel H, et al. Dual time-point FDG PET-CT for differentiating benign from malignant solitary pulmonary nodules in a TB endemic area. S Afr Med J 2010;100:598–601.
10. Chen CJ, Lee BF, Yao WJ, et al. ·Dual-phase 18F-FDG PET in the diagnosis of pulmonary nodules with an initial standard uptake value less than 2.5. AJR Am J Roentgenol 2008;191:475–9.
11. Shim SS, Lee KS, Kim BT, et al. Non-small cell lung cancer: prospective comparison of integrated FDG PET/CT and CT alone for preoperative staging. Radiology 2005;236:1011–9.
12. Haroon A, Zumla A, Bomanji J. Role of fluorine 18 fluorodeoxyglucose positron emission tomography-computed tomography in focal and generalized infectious and inflammatory disorders. Clin Infect Dis 2012;54:1333–41.
13. Kim IJ, Lee JS, Kim SJ, et al. Double-phase 18F-FDG PET-CT for determination of pulmonary tuberculoma activity. Eur J Nucl Med Mol Imaging 2008;35:808–14.
14. Siegel R, Ward E, Brawley O, et al. Cancer statistics, 2011: the impact of eliminating socioeconomic and racial disparities on premature cancer deaths. CA Cancer J Clin 2011;61:212–36.
15. Frieden TR. The health consequences of smoking-50 years of progress. A report of the Surgeon General. Atlanta (GA): US Department of Health and Human services; 2014. p. 143–7.
16. Secretan B, Straif K, Baan R, et al. A review of human carcinogens–Part E: tobacco, areca nut, alcohol, coal smoke, and salted fish. Lancet Oncol 2009;10:1033–4.
17. Doll R, Peto R. Mortality in relation to smoking: 20 years' observations on male British doctors. Br Med J 1976;2(6051):1525–36.
18. Omenn GS, Merchant J, Boatman E, et al. Contribution of environmental fibers to respiratory cancer. Environ Health Perspect 1986;70:51–6.
19. Taylor R, Najafi F, Dobson A. Meta-analysis of studies of passive smoking and lung cancer: effects of study type and continent. Int J Epidemiol 2007;36(5):1048–59.
20. Wald NJ, Nanchahal K, Thompson SG, et al. Does breathing other people's tobacco smoke cause lung cancer? Br Med J 1986;293(6556):1217–22 (Clin Res Ed).
21. Cegielski JP, Chin DP, Espinal MA, et al. The global tuberculosis situation: progress and problems in the 20th century, prospects for the 21st century. Infect Dis Clin North Am 2002;16:1–58.
22. Corbett EL, Watt CJ, Walker N, et al. The growing burden of tuberculosis: global trends and interactions with the HIV epidemic. Arch Intern Med 2003;163:1009–21.
23. Tufariello JM, Chan J, Flynn JL. Latent tuberculosis: mechanisms of host and bacillus that contribute to persistent infection. Lancet Infect Dis 2003;3:578–90.
24. World Health Organization. Global tuberculosis report. Geneva (Switzeland): World health Organization; 2013.
25. Zumla A, Ravigliona M, Hafner R, et al. Tuberculosis. N Engl J Med 2013;368:745–55.
26. Jeong YJ, Lee KS. Pulmonary tuberculosis: up-to date imaging and management. AJR Am J Roentgenol 2008;191:834–44.
27. Sochocky S. Tuberculoma of the lung. Am Rev Tuberc 1958;78:403–10.
28. Houben EN, Nguyen L, Pieters J. Interaction of pathogenic mycobacteria with the host immune system. Curr Opin Microbiol 2006;9:76–85.
29. Kaufmann SH. Protection against tuberculosis: cytokines, T cells, and macrophages. Ann Rheum Dis 2002;61(Suppl 2):ii54–8.
30. Alavi A, Gupta N, Alberini JL, et al. Positron emission tomography imaging in nonmalignant thoracic disorders. Semin Nucl Med 2002;32:293–321.

31. Kubota R, Yamada S, Kubota K, et al. Intra tumoral distribution of fluorine-18-fluorodeoxyglucose in vivo: high accumulation macrophages and granulation tissues studied by microautoradiography. J Nucl Med 1992;33:1972–80.

32. Mochizuki T, Tsukamoto E, Kuge Y, et al. FDG uptake and glucose transporter subtype expression in experimental tumor and inflammation models. J Nucl Med 2001;42:1551–5.

33. Paik JY, Lee KH, Choe YS, et al. Augmented 18F-FDG uptake in activated monocytes occurs during the priming process and involves tyrosine kinases and protein kinase C. J Nucl Med 2004;45:124–8.

34. Zhuang H, Alavi A. 18-Florodeoxyglucose positron emission tomography imaging in the detection and monitoring of infection. and inflammation. Semin Nucl Med 2002;32:47–59.

35. Fischer BM, Mortensen J. The future in diagnosis and staging of lung cancer: positron emission tomography. Respiration 2006;73:267–76.

36. Kuehl H, Veit P, Rosenbaum SJ, et al. Can PET/CT replace separate diagnostic CT for cancer imaging? Optimizing CT protocols for imaging cancers of the chest and abdomen. J Nucl Med 2007;48(Suppl 1):45S–57S.

37. Lowe VJ, Hoffman JM, DeLong DM, et al. Semiquantitative and visual analysis of 18F-FDG PET images in pulmonary abnormalities. J Nucl Med 1994;35:1771–6.

38. Gupta N, Gill H, Graeber G, et al. Dynamic positron emission tomography with 18F-fluorodeoxyglucose imaging in differentiation of benign from malignant lung/mediastinal lesions. Chest 1998;114:1105–11.

39. Gupta NC, Maloof J, Gunel E. Probability of malignancy in solitary pulmonary nodules using 18F-FDG and PET. J Nucl Med 1996;37:943–8.

40. Yang SN, Liang JA, Lin FJ, et al. Differentiating benign and malignant pulmonary lesions with 18F-FDG PET. Anticancer Res 2001;21:4153–7.

41. Dobaylongod FG, Lowe VJ, Patz EF Jr, et al. Detection of primary and recurrent lung cancer by means of 18F fluorodeoxyglucose positron emission tomography (18F-FDG PET). J Thorac Cardiovasc Surg 1995;110:130–9.

42. Lindell RM, Hartman TE, Swensen SJ, et al. Lung cancer screening experience: a retrospective review of PET in 22 non-small cell lung carcinomas detected on screening chest CT in a high-risk population. AJR Am J Roentgenol 2005;185:126–31.

43. Shon IH, O'Doherty MJ, Maisey MN. Positron emission tomography in lung cancer. Semin Nucl Med 2002;32:240–71.

44. Fischer BM, Mortensen J, Hojaard L. PET in the diagnosis and staging of lung cancer-a systematic, quantitative review of the literature. Lancet Oncol 2001;2:659–66.

45. Gould MK, Maclean CC, Kuschner WG, et al. Accuracy of positron emission tomography for diagnosis of pulmonary nodules and mass lesions: a meta-analysis. JAMA 2001;285:914–24.

46. Groft DR, Trapp J, Kemstine K, et al. 18F-FDG PET imaging and the diagnosis of non-small cell lung cancer in region of high histoplasmosis prevalence. Lung Cancer 2002;36:297–301.

47. Via LE, Schimel D, Weiner DM, et al. Infection dynamics and response to chemotherapy in rabbit model of tuberculosis using 18F-fluoro-deoxy-D-glucose positron emission tomography and computed tomography. Antimicrob Agents Chemother 2012;56:4391–402.

48. Lin PL, Ford CB, Coleman MT, et al. Sterilization of granulomas is common in both active and inactive tuberculosis despite extensive within-host variability in bacterial killing. Nat Med 2014;20:75–9.

49. Coleman MT, Maiello P, Tomko J, et al. Early changes by 18F fluorodeoxyglucose positron emission tomography coregistered with computed tomography predict outcome after mycobacterium tuberculosis infection in cynomolgus macaques. Infect Immun 2014;82:2400–4.

50. Low SY, Eng P, Keng GH, et al. Positron emission tomography with CT in the evaluation of non-small cell lung cancer in population with a high prevalence of tuberculosis. Respirology 2006;11:84–9.

51. Harkirat S, Anand SS, Indrajit IK, et al. Pictorial essay: PET/CT in tuberculosis. Indian J Radiol Imaging 2008;18:141–7.

52. Yang CM, Hsu CH, Lee CM, et al. Intense uptake of 18F-fluoro-2deoxy-D-glucose in active pulmonary tuberculosis. Ann Nucl Med 2003;17:407–10.

53. Goo JM, Im JG, Do KH, et al. Pulmonary tuberculoma evaluated by means of FDG PET: findings in 10 cases. Radiology 2000;216:117–21.

54. Matthies A, Hickeson M, Cuchiara A, et al. Dual time point 18F-FDG PET for the evaluation of pulmonary nodules. J Nucl Med 2002;43:871–5.

55. Xiu Y, Bhutani C, Dhurairaj T, et al. Dual-time point FDG PET imaging in the evaluation of pulmonary nodules with minimally increased metabolic activity. Clin Nucl Med 2007;32:101–5.

56. Alkhawaldeh K, Bural G, Kumar R, et al. Impact of dual-time point (18) F-FDG-PET imaging in partial volume correction in the assessment of pulmonary solitary nodules. Eur J Nucl Med Mol Imaging 2008;35:246–52.

57. Macdonald K, Saerle J, Lyburn I. The role of dual time point FDG PET imaging in the evaluation of solitary pulmonary nodules with an initial standard uptake value less than 2.5. Clin Radiol 2011;66:244–50.

58. Yang P, Xu YY, Liu XJ, et al. The value of delayed (18) F-FDG-PET imaging in diagnosing of solitary

pulmonary nodules: a preliminary study on 28 patients. Quant Imaging Med Surg 2011;1:31–4.

59. Lan XL, Zhang YW, Wu ZJ, et al. The value of dual time point (18)F-FDG PET imaging for the differentiation between malignant and benign lesions. Clin Radiol 2008;63:756–64.

60. Hamberg LM, Hunter GJ, Alpert NM, et al. The dose uptake ratio as an index of glucose metabolism: useful parameter or oversimplification? J Nucl Med 1994;35:1308–12.

61. Laffon E, de Clermont H, Begueret H, et al. Assessment of dual-time 18F-FDG PET in the diagnosis of pulmonary lesions. Nucl Med Commun 2009;30:455–61.

62. Deppen S, Putnam JB Jr, Andrade G, et al. Accuracy of FDG-PET to diagnose lung cancer in region of endemic granulomatous disease. Ann Thorac Surg 2011;92:428–33.

63. Bleeker-Rovers CP, Vos FJ, Corstens FH, et al. Imaging of infectious disease using [¹⁸F] fluorodeoxyglucose PET. Q J Nucl Med Mol Imaging 2008;52:17–29.

64. Bryant AS, Cerfolio RJ. The maximum standardized uptake values on integrated FDG PET/CT are useful in differentiating benign from malignant pulmonary nodules. Ann Thorac Surg 2006;82:1016–20.

65. Hot A, Maunoury C, Poiree S, et al. Diagnostic contribution of positron emission tomography with [¹⁸F] fluorodeoxyglucose for invasive fungal infection. Clin Microbiol Infect 2011;17:409–17.

66. Prabhakar HB, Rabinowitz CB, Gibbons FK, et al. Imaging features of sarcoidosis on MDCT, FDG PET and PET/CT. AJR Am J Roentgenol 2008;190(3 suppl):S1–6.

67. Yamada Y, Uchida Y, Tatsumi K, et al. Fluorine-18-fluorodeoxyglucose and carbon-11-methionine evaluation of lymphadenopathy in sarcoidosis. J Nucl Med 1998;39:1160–6.

68. Braun JJ, Kessler R, Constantinesco A, et al. 18F-FDG PET/CT in sarcoidosis management: review and report of 20 cases. Eur J Nucl Med Mol Imaging 2008;35:1537–43.

69. Keijisers RG, Verzijlbergen FJ, Oyen WJ, et al. 18F-FDG-PET, genotype-corrected ACE and siL2R in newly diagnosed sarcoidosis. Eur J Nucl Med Mol Imaging 2009;36:1131–7.

70. Keijisers RG, Grutters JC, Thomeer M, et al. Imaging the inflammatory activity of sarcoidosis; sensitivity and inter observer agreement of (67)Ga imaging and (18)F-FDG PET. Q J Nucl Med Imaging 2011;55:66–71.

71. Lequoy M, Coriat R, Rouguette A, et al. Sarcoidosis lung nodules in colorectal cancer follow-up: sarcoidosis or not? Am J Med 2013;126:642–5.

72. Koyama T, Ueda H, Togashi K, et al. Radiologic manifestations of sarcoidosis in various organs. Radiographics 2004;24:87–104.

73. Lim JH, Lee JH. Inflammatory pseudotumor of liver: ultrasound and CT features. Clin Imaging 1995;19:43–6.

74. Kelekis NL, Warshauer DM, Semelka RC, et al. Inflammatory pseudotumor of the liver: appearance on contrast enhanced helical CT and dynamic MR images. J Magn Reson Imaging 1995;5:551–3.

75. Huellner MW, Schwizer B, Burger I, et al. Inflammatory pseudotumor of lung with high FDG uptake. Clin Nucl Med 2010;35:722–3.

76. Zheng Z, Pan Y, Pan T, et al. Coexistent pulmonary inflammatory pseudotumor and carcinoma in one patient: does positron emission tomography/computed tomography help. Ann Thorac Surg 2011;91:e43.

77. Hirose Y, Kaida H, Kurata S, et al. Incidental detection of rare mesenteric inflammatory pseudotumor by (18)F-FDG PET. Hell J Nucl Med 2012;15:247–50.

78. Lee JH, Lee KG, Park HK, et al. Inflammatory pseudotumor of the kidney mimicking malignancy on 18F-FDG PET/CT in a patient with diabetes and hepatocellular carcinoma. Clin Nucl Med 2012;37:699–701.

79. Huang YE, Huang YJ, Ko M, et al. Dual-time-point 18F-FDG PET/CT in the diagnosis of solitary pulmonary lesions in a region with endemic granulomatous. Ann Nucl Med 2016;30:652–8.

80. Chen S, Li X, Chen M, et al. Limited diagnostic value of dual-time-point (18)F-FDG PET/CT imaging for classifying solitary pulmonary nodules in granuloma-endemic regions both at visual and quantitative analyses. Eur J Radiol 2016;85:1744–9.

Genomic Characterization of Lung Cancer and Its Impact on the Use and Timing of PET in Therapeutic Response Assessment

CrossMark

Lavinia Tan, MBBS, FRACP[a],
Benjamin Solomon, MBBS, PhD, FRACP[a,b],*

KEYWORDS

- Genomics • Non–small cell lung cancer (NSCLC) • PET • Therapeutic response assessment

KEY POINTS

- Non–small cell lung cancer (NSCLC) is a heterogeneous disease comprising different histologic and molecular subtypes with distinct clinical characteristics, outcomes, and prognosis.
- PET has an established role in the diagnosis, staging, and monitoring of therapeutic response in patients with NSCLC.
- Early therapeutic response on PET is associated with improved outcomes in patients receiving targeted therapies.
- Newer PET tracers have been developed in hopes of improving the sensitivity and specificity of PET imaging in predicting response to therapeutic targets.

INTRODUCTION

Lung cancer remains one of the leading causes of cancer-related mortality, with most patients presenting with locally advanced or metastatic disease.[1] The widespread implementation of ^{18}F-fluorodeoxyglucose (FDG) PET has led to earlier diagnosis of lung cancer with a more accurate assessment of nodal and distant metastatic disease, leading to improvements in treatment planning and selection.[2] Imaging in tumor response assessment is central in determining therapeutic decisions for individual patients as well as quantifying benefit of novel therapies in clinical trials.

In this review article, the authors summarize the genomic landscape of non–small cell lung cancer (NSCLC), highlighting genotypes with available targeted therapies and the implication of clonal evolution and intratumor heterogeneity in the development of drug resistance. They review the impact and timing of PET in therapeutic response assessment in NSCLC, together with limitations of conventional response assessment criteria in the era of targeted therapies and immunotherapies. Also discussed are emerging PET radiotracers that have been developed and evaluated as a noninvasive assessment of biological processes in vivo.

Disclosure Statement: No relevant conflicts of interest.
[a] Department of Medical Oncology, Peter MacCallum Cancer Centre, 305 Grattan Street, Melbourne, Victoria 3000, Australia; [b] Sir Peter MacCallum Department of Oncology, University of Melbourne, Grattan Street, Parkville, Victoria 3052, Australia
* Corresponding author. Peter MacCallum Cancer Centre, 305 Grattan Street, Melbourne, Victoria 3000, Australia.
E-mail address: ben.solomon@petermac.org

PET Clin 13 (2018) 33–42
http://dx.doi.org/10.1016/j.cpet.2017.08.004
1556-8598/18/© 2017 Elsevier Inc. All rights reserved.

THE GENOMIC LANDSCAPE OF NON–SMALL CELL LUNG CANCER

NSCLC accounts for 85% of all lung cancer cases and comprises 3 major histologic subtypes with the most common being adenocarcinoma followed by squamous cell carcinoma and less commonly large cell carcinoma.[1] Most cases of lung cancer are related to tobacco smoking; however, approximately 10% to 20% of cases occur in patients who have never smoked, and the declining rates of smoking equals a proportional increase of incidence among never smokers.[3,4] Smoking-related lung cancer has a significantly higher number of mutations and is associated with cytosine to adenine (C > A) nucleotide transversions. Transversions have been associated with different gene mutations in lung cancer; for example, KRAS mutations are more frequent in transversion high patients, compared with transversion low patients, who are commonly never smokers and have a higher prevalence of EGFR mutations.[3,5]

In the last decade or so, the application of more advanced and accurate high-throughput platform with next-generation sequencing has led to the first genome-wide mutational analyses.[5,6] Lung adenocarcinoma has high rates of somatic mutation, and it is possible to identify oncogenic driver mutations in more than 50% of cases.[7] Driver mutations initiate the transformation of a nonmalignant cell to malignancy and sustain the tumor's survival. This concept of "oncogene addiction," which makes the tumor extremely reliant on downstream growth and survival pathways, provides a potential molecular Achilles heel that may be targeted therapeutically.[8,9]

The most frequent oncogenic driver mutations in lung adenocarcinoma include KRAS mutations (33% of tumors), EGFR mutations (15%), ALK rearrangements (3%–5%), BRAF mutations (2%), ROS1 rearrangements (1%–2%), PIK3CA mutations (1%–2%), and MET amplifications (1%–2%) (**Fig. 1**). Several other common, but not clinically actionable, loss-of-function mutations and deletions in tumor suppressor genes are as follows: TP53 (46% of tumors), STK11 (17%), RB1 (4%), NF1 (11%), CDKN2A (4%), SMARCA4 (10%), and KEAP1 (17%). In recent years, molecular targeted therapies have improved the outcome of patients whose tumors harbor an activating mutation in EGFR or ALK and ROS1 gene rearrangement, with other investigational therapies targeting BRAF, MET, and RET currently in clinical trials.[5,7,10]

Squamous cell lung carcinomas are characterized by a high overall mutation rate and marked genomic complexity. Compared with adenocarcinoma, almost all squamous cell lung cancers display somatic mutation of TP53, with fewer mutations in genes encoding receptor tyrosine kinase and a higher frequency of loss of tumor suppressor functions affecting genes such as PTEN, NOTCH1, and RB1.[11] Potential therapeutic targets have been identified, such as FGFR1 amplification, DDR2 mutation, and PIK3CA amplification and mutation, with preliminary activity seen in some early phase trials.[12–14] Although the genomic landscape of NSCLC is illustrated by large numbers of somatic copy number alteration, gene rearrangement, and recurrent alteration in multiple key pathways, most patients lack an actionable driver mutation and are therefore treated with nontargeted therapies, such as chemotherapy or immunotherapy.

At present, structural imaging with computed tomographic (CT) scan is still the standard diagnostic imaging test for assessing therapeutic response, in either the curative setting or more advanced disease. There are, however, several limitations with structural imaging in NSCLC that impede the ability to accurately assess response, including (1) difficulty of CT scan in differentiating between tumor and inflammation or scar tissue after surgery or radiotherapy; (2) difficulty measuring irregular tumor shapes; (3) inaccuracy of lymph node staging; (4) consolidation of the lung obscuring tumors; and (5) poor contrast enhancement between tumor and normal thoracic structures.[15]

PET/CT is becoming the new standard of care in the diagnosis and staging of NSCLC given its high diagnostic accuracy. It provides a more comprehensive assessment of both structural and biological changes[16–18] and is increasingly being used for monitoring treatment response.

Genotypes with Available Targeted Therapies

The discoveries of oncogenic drivers together with the development of targeted therapies have revolutionized the management of advanced NSCLC, improving outcomes for the subgroup of patients with actionable molecular targets. The Lung Cancer Mutation Consortium demonstrated that patients with actionable oncogenic driver mutations who were treated with molecular targeted therapies lived longer.[7] Current guidelines from the College of American Pathologist, International Association for the Study of Lung Cancer, and Association for Molecular Pathology recommend testing for EGFR mutation and ALK rearrangement in all patients with advanced stage

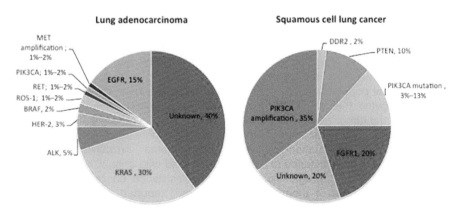

Fig. 1. Relative frequency of genomic alterations in lung adenocarcinoma and squamous cell lung carcinoma. *ALK*, anaplastic lymphoma kinase; *BRAF*, B-raf proto-oncogene; *DDR2*, discoidin death receptor 2; *EGFR*, epidermal growth factor receptor; *FGFR1*, fibroblast growth factor 1; *HER-2*, human epidermal growth receptor 2; *KRAS*, Kirsten rat sarcoma virus; *MET*, MET proto-oncogene; *PIK3CA*, phosphatidylinositol 3-kinase; *PTEN*, phosphatase and tensin homolog deleted on chromosome 10; *RET*, ret proto-oncogene; *ROS1*, ROS proto-oncogene 1.

adenocarcinoma, regardless of clinical characteristics of the patient.[19]

Activating *EGFR* mutations are key drivers in NSCLC in approximately 10% to 15% of Western patients and 30% to 35% of Asian patients.[20] The clinically relevant and most frequent *EGFR* mutations are in-frame deletions/insertions of exon 19 (40%–50%) and L858R mutation of exon 21 (30%–40%); both associated with sensitivity to EGFR tyrosine kinase inhibitors (TKIs). First- and second-generation EGFR TKIs, gefitinib, erlotinib, and afatinib, have been shown in 7 randomized phase 3 trials to improve progression-free survival (PFS), objective response rate (ORR), and quality of life of patients with *EGFR* mutation-positive NSCLC over standard first-line doublet chemotherapy. With the exception of patients with *EGFR* exon 19 deletion treated with afatinib in both the LUX-Lung 3 and the LUX-Lung 6 trials, an overall survival advantage has not been clearly demonstrated in trials involving gefitinib or erlotinib due to crossover designs confounding survival data.[21–28]

ALK gene rearrangements occur in 3% to 5% of NSCLC patients, with a higher frequency in adenocarcinomas, never or light smokers, and younger patients.[29,30] Crizotinib, an oral, small-molecule TKI of ALK, MET, and ROS1 kinases, was shown to have superior response rates and prolonged PFS over standard chemotherapy, establishing it as standard first-line treatment of newly diagnosed patients with advanced *ALK* rearranged NSCLC.[31] Recently, a second-generation ALK TKI ceritinib was shown to be superior to chemotherapy in a phase 3 trial (ASCEND-4), in ALK inhibitor-naïve patients, providing an additional option for first-line therapy.[32]

Implications of Clonal Evolution and Intratumor Heterogeneity in Drug Resistance

The accumulation of genetic alterations and the selective pressure that favors the growth and survival of subpopulations of somatic cells with a biological advantage underlie the genetic evolution that gives rise to cancer. The most important mutations are "driver mutations," which are critical to cancer development and maintenance, whereas "passenger mutations" do not confer a growth advantage.[33] It has been postulated that the role of somatic mutations as "driver" or "passenger" may vary, subject to environmental and treatment selection pressures, whereby passengers may become drivers and vice versa.[34] There is now evidence that tumors are genetically heterogenous, with the potential for distinct subclones to evolve throughout the disease process. It is therefore important to obtain an accurate view of this dynamic genomic landscape in order to choose the correct therapeutic regimen.[35]

Tumor heterogeneity refers to the presence of subclonal population with different genotypes and associated phenotypes mixed within a primary tumor, between primary and its metastases or between metastatic sites. One of the major challenges of intratumor heterogeneity lies in the fact that sampling of a single region at the time of biopsy may not capture the complete spectrum of mutations within a tumor. Furthermore, genomic analyses have recently revealed molecular evidence of branched tumor evolution, whereby tumors consist of distinct subclones evolving in parallel resulting in subclonal diversity.[4,36] The fluctuations in subclonal populations can occur, for example, with therapy or during metastatic disease progression, leading to a selective outgrowth of clones that best adapt to the tumor microenvironment.[33,34]

It has been reported that resistance to targeted therapies can result from the outgrowth of preexisting subclonal populations that confer resistance to the targeted therapy, which may have been present in the tumor at low frequency before treatment initiation. As an example, 50% to 70% of patients with *EGFR* mutation-positive NSCLC will ultimately develop resistance to first- or second-generation TKI with progression of disease after 9 to 13 months of therapy.[37,38] Acquired resistance to TKIs can come about through various mechanisms with the most common one due to T790M "gatekeeper" mutation in approximately 50% to 60% of cases.[39,40] With more sensitive sequencing technologies, it has been discovered that existing *EGFR*-T790M clones can be detected at low frequencies in patients who are TKI naïve.[41] The selection of preexisting *EGFR*-T790M-positive clones under pressure from an EGFR TKI explains the emergence of resistance in this instance, highlighting tumor heterogeneity and adaptability.[42]

Osimertinib is an oral, potent, irreversible EGFR TKI selective for T790M resistance mutation and *EGFR* sensitizing mutations, while sparing the activity of wild-type *EGFR*.[43] Most recently, data from a phase 3 trial (AURA-3) established osimertinib as a superior treatment over chemotherapy in the second-line setting after failure of an earlier generation EGFR-TKI therapy in patients whose tumors are positive for T790M mutation.[44] However, with selection pressure, resistance to third-generation EGFR TKI ultimately develops. In a study performed by Thress and colleagues[45] on cell-free plasma DNA of patients whose tumor developed resistance to osimertinib, various mechanisms of resistance have been identified with the most frequent one being the acquisition of *EGFR*-C797S mutation in exon 20 of *EGFR*. Other mechanisms of resistance that have been described include loss of T790M mutation after treatment with osimertinib and concurrent acquired C797S mutations, highlighting the genomic heterogeneity of *EGFR* mutant NSCLC.

Mechanisms of Drug Resistance in ALK Rearranged Non–Small Cell Lung Cancer

Unlike EGFR TKI resistance, there is a greater diversity of molecular mechanisms of ALK inhibitor resistance involving on-target genetic alterations (eg, *ALK* resistance mutations, *ALK* gene amplification)

in about one-third of patients progressing on crizotinib, or off-target mechanisms of resistance (eg, upregulation of bypass signaling pathways: EGFR, KIT, MEK/ERK, and others).[46] Newer-generation ALK inhibitors including ceretinib, alectinib, and brigatinib have been shown to have impressive activity in not only patients progressing on crizotinib but also crizotinib-naïve patients. In addition, these agents are more potent and have been developed to overcome crizotinib resistance variably. Compared with only 20% of patients who developed resistance on crizotinib, Gainor and colleagues[46] reported a different spectrum of *ALK* resistance mutations present in more than half of patients progressing on second-generation ALK inhibitors. As resistance evolves over time and develops in response to sequential ALK inhibitors, the management of *ALK* rearranged NSCLC becomes more complex. It is therefore crucial to identify resistance early on to allow clinicians to select the most effective therapeutic strategy for the patient.

RESPONSE ASSESSMENT CRITERIA IN LUNG CANCER

Early and robust evaluation of tumor response in lung cancer is needed to avoid unnecessary side effects of ineffective treatment and delay switching to a more efficacious alternative therapy.[2,47] Multiple guidelines have been developed to assess therapeutic response in clinical trials as a potential surrogate for survival, such as the World Health Organization (WHO) criteria (1979), Response Evaluation Criteria in Solid Tumors (RECIST) 2000, and RECIST 1.1 (2009). RECIST criteria, a modification of the earlier WHO response criteria, assesses tumor response based on percentage change in tumor lesions measured over time as identified on CT scan and is defined by complete response, partial response, stable disease and progressive disease. Changes in tumor size after treatment are often, but not always, related to therapeutic efficacy and have been shown to be predictive of survival.[48] In a meta-analysis performed by Blumenthal and colleagues[49] using both trial and patient entry level data from 14 clinical trials, including 3 smaller randomized studies involving *ALK* rearrangement or *EGFR* mutation-positive patients, a strong association was found between overall response rate and PFS, with no association found between overall survival (OS) and ORR or OS and PFS. Hence, therapies with significant ORRs are a strong predictor of clinical benefit and would likely have a large impact on PFS.

Limitations of Conventional Response Assessment Criteria in Lung Cancer

There are limitations to conventional tumor response assessment in lung cancer, such as (1) difficulty measuring true tumor size because tumor may comprise malignant cells, stroma, and inflammatory cells; (2) confounding effects of atelectasis, radiation pneumonitis, and posttreatment fibrosis[2]; (3) unidimensional measurements may not capture lesions with asymmetrical growth patterns; (4) tumor cavitation is commonly observed after radiotherapy and EGFR TKIs in lung cancer, making it difficult to measure accurately; (5) underestimation of therapeutic activity of molecular targeted therapies that works via inhibition of cell proliferation; (6) progression by RECIST may not warrant a change in treatment in the era of molecular targeted therapies and immunotherapies.[50,51]

Metabolic Response Criteria

With an increasing move toward using PET/CT in therapeutic response assessment, the European Organization for Research and Treatment of Cancer (EORTC) guidelines were developed in 1999 as a common measurement standard criteria for reporting alterations in [^{18}F]-FDG uptake to assess clinical and subclinical response.[52] The best known parameter to measure response is the standardized uptake value (SUV), which is derived by dividing the measured radioactivity in tissue by the total activity administered to the patient and the patient's weight after correcting for various factors, whereas the maximum SUV (SUV_{max}) in a lesion is the most reproducible parameter and has therefore become the preferred parameter for assessing therapeutic response.[2] It has previously been shown that a reduction in SUV after one cycle of chemotherapy ($15\% \pm 30\%$) can predict clinical response that precedes tumor shrinkage.[52]

The EORTC defines an objective PET response (partial metabolic response) as an SUV_{max} decrease of greater than 15% after one cycle of chemotherapy or greater than 25% after more than one treatment cycle. PET stable metabolic disease was defined as mean change of 0% to 15% in SUV_{max}, and PET progressive metabolic disease was defined as the mean increase of greater than 15% or one or more new metastatic lesions on PET. A complete metabolic response would be complete resolution of ^{18}F-FDG uptake within the tumor volume indistinguishable from surrounding normal tissue.[52]

In 2009, Wahl and colleagues[48] proposed the Positron Emission Tomography Response Criteria In Solid Tumors (PERCIST) 1.0 criteria on the premise that tumor response as assessed by PET is a continuous and time-dependent variable. It is a quantitative assessment of metabolic changes in tumor at different time points, providing a more accurate and early therapeutic response assessment. With PERCIST, a single target lesion with the highest metabolic activity is selected at each time point, reflecting the most aggressive site of disease. SUV corrected for lean body mass (SUL) is determined for up to 5 lesions at baseline, and the SUL_{peak} is measured in the single hottest tumor. This is identified manually by moving a fixed 1-mL spherical volume of interest and finding the focus of tumor with the highest mean SUL value. Response assessment as per PERCIST 1.0 is based on the percentage change in SUL_{peak} between pretreatment and posttreatment scans. Although functional imaging with ^{18}F-FDG PET is increasingly being used as an early assessment of treatment, there is still no consensus on the preferred methodology, measurement parameters, and response definition.

Immune-Related Response Criteria

Immunotherapy has emerged as a principal therapeutic modality for patients with advanced NSCLC. The results from KEYNOTE-024 randomized trial have established pembrolizumab, a monoclonal antibody against programmed death-1 (PD-1), as first-line treatment over standard platinum doublet chemotherapy for advanced NSCLC with PD-L1 expression of at least 50% of tumor cells.[53] In addition, Nivolumab has been shown to have a significantly better OS, response rate, and PFS over chemotherapy in the second-line setting for patients with advanced NSCLC.[54,55] Immune-related response criteria (irRC) was developed to fully characterize and assess atypical response patterns in this new era of immunotherapeutic agents. The irRC recognizes that the appearance of anti-tumor activity may take longer for immunotherapy compared with conventional chemotherapy; atypical responses may occur termed "pseudoprogression" due to inflammatory cell infiltration or necrosis, and durable stable disease can be an indicator of anti-tumor activity.[50] Key differences between RECIST and irRC include the incorporation of measurable new lesions into the "total tumor burden," whereas new lesions on RECIST would define disease progression.

Beyond ^{18}F-Fluorodeoxyglucose: Newer PET Tracers

The most widely used radiotracer ^{18}F-FDG, a glucose analogue, is transported into cells by the sodium-independent glucose transporter proteins (GLUT-1), which is commonly expressed in NSCLC. FDG is phosphorylated by hexokinase and trapped intracellularly, accumulating in malignant cells due to the increased rate of glucose metabolism in tumor cells.[56–59] The extent and levels of expression of GLUT-1 has been shown to correlate with high FDG uptake.[60] Preclinical studies have confirmed that AKT, the downstream serine-threonine kinase of EGFR signaling, plays an important role in cell survival of *EGFR* mutant NSCLC through exerting a direct influence on glycolysis by several mechanisms, such as the initiation of GLUT-1 synthesis, the translocation of glucose transporters from plasma membrane to the cytosol, and upregulation of hexokinase and phosphofructokinase activity.[58,59,61] The inhibition of AKT through EGFR TKIs erlotinib and gefitinib leads to the downregulation of GLUT-1 expression in sensitive cells, causing marked reduction of glucose utilization, resulting in apoptosis and subsequent morphologic regression.[47,57,62] However, ^{18}F-FDG is not highly specific for malignancy and is also taken up by inflammatory cells, such as macrophages and granulation tissue.[63,64]

Beyond glucose metabolism, other biological functions can be tested, including hypoxia, amino acid metabolism, angiogenesis, and proliferation. [^{18}F]-Fluoro-L-thymidine ([^{18}F] FLT), a radiolabeled form of pyrimidine nucleoside, is transported into cells and phosphorylated by thymidine kinase 1 (TK1). [^{18}F]FLT signal detected by PET provides a reasonable measure of cellular TK1 activity, which acts as a surrogate marker of tumor cell proliferation.[64–66] Moreover, Buck and colleagues[67] have shown that [18]FLT uptake, which is exclusively present in malignant lesions, is highly correlated with Ki-67 immunostaining, a marker of proliferative activity. Barthel and colleagues[65] have also shown a more pronounced decrease in [^{18}F]FLT compared with FDG after 1 week of chemotherapy, making it a sensitive marker of tumor response to therapy. These promising data will need to be assessed in additional prospective studies to evaluate FLT PET as an alternative to FDG PET in assessing response in NSCLC.

More recently, promising and emerging radiolabeled anticancer agents have been developed to quantify therapeutic targets and assess drug concentration in vivo. Binding of radiolabeled anticancer agents to tumor can predict drug sensitivity and early detection of molecular resistance.[68] So far, these have been used in the research setting with limited clinical utility. Of interest to NSCLC, [11C]-erlotinib was developed by Memon and colleagues and was shown to accumulate in xenografts that were sensitive to erlotinib treatment and expressed high levels of EGFR. In a study of 13 patients with NSCLC, [11C]-erlotinib PET identified both enlarged and nonenlarged lymph nodes that were negative on FDG-PET, suggesting a more sensitive method of lymph node staging in these patients. In addition, different accumulation of [11C]-erlotinib was observed between different tumors in the same patient, suggesting tumor heterogeneity. Nevertheless, larger clinical studies would be required to verify the efficacy of [11C]-erlotinib PET in predicting response to treatment.[69,70]

The use of FDG PET to assess response to immunotherapy has been challenging given that both tumor and immune infiltrates can be FDG-avid, making it difficult to differentiate between progression and "pseudoprogression." PD-L1, an immune checkpoint protein expressed on tumor cells and tumor-infiltrating immune cells, is expressed in a wide variety of tumors, including NSCLC. Atezolizumab, a humanized immunoglobulin G1 monoclonal antibody targeting PD-L1, has been shown in a phase 3 randomized trial to be superior to chemotherapy in previously treated NSCLC patients.[71] Molecular imaging with PET using zirconium-89 ([89]Zr) -radiolabeled atezolizumab is currently being trialed clinically as a new tracer in breast cancer, bladder cancer, and NSCLC.[72] It has a potential role in identifying patients who will benefit the most from checkpoint blockade therapy by detecting PD-L1 expression in tumors and distinguishing between radiographic "pseudoprogression" and progression. The emergence of these novel tracers has further defined the potential role of PET as a prognostic and predictive biomarker in the treatment of lung cancer.

Timing of PET in Therapeutic Response Assessment in Lung Cancer

Early detection of recurrence after curative therapy for NSCLC is essential as localized relapse may be cured with appropriate aggressive therapy. In a prospective study, Mac Manus and colleagues[15] reported that a single, early, posttreatment PET scan is a better predictor of survival than CT response. It was also suggested that PET response could be used to determine the benefit of further therapy after chemoradiation in patients with locoregionally persistent disease. Furthermore, preliminary data demonstrated a reduced rate of subsequent distant metastasis in patients with a PET complete response; however, longer follow-up is needed in this group of patients.

It has been established that EGFR signaling pathways have a role in regulating tumor glucose metabolism, making ^{18}F-FDG PET a good modality for monitoring treatment response in *EGFR* mutation-positive NSCLC. Furthermore, a more rapid change in cellular metabolism compared with a decrease in tumor size makes treatment-induced changes as measured by a reduction in FDG or FLT uptake by PET a sensitive technique of assessment and an early marker of response.[73,74]

Several preclinical studies in NSCLC have evaluated ^{18}F-FDG and [^{18}F]FLT PET as an early marker of response to TKIs. Su and colleagues[57] demonstrated a rapid reduction in FDG uptake after only 48 hours of EGFR TKI in gefitinib-sensitive cell lines, while Ullrich and colleagues[66] showed that using [^{18}F] FLT PET was more accurate than FDG PET in detecting a response in mice receiving erlotinib treatment as early as 48 hours after the onset of treatment. This was also shown clinically by Sunaga and colleagues,[74] who demonstrated a rapid response to gefitinib therapy as early as 2 days in 5 patients, as measured by a reduction in FDG uptake. Sohn and colleagues[75] found that early changes in [^{18}F]FLT PET after 7 days of gefitinib predicted response to treatment in non-smokers with advanced adenocarcinoma of the lung. A review by van Gool and colleagues[76] showed a large variation in days (2–56 days) between initiation of EGFR TKI therapy and response on PET with informative results as early as 7 to 14 days.

Both Mileshkin and colleagues[62] and Zander and colleagues[77] have shown that early FDG PET and [^{18}F]FLT PET response (day 14 and day 7, respectively) is associated with longer OS in patients receiving EGFR TKIs. Similarly, Soto-Para and colleagues[78] reported that patients with an early metabolic response have better outcomes with longer PFS and OS. In addition, Tiseo and colleagues[47] found that all patients with early metabolic progressive disease on FDG PET assessment after 2 days of erlotinib had significantly shorter survival. Takahashi and colleagues,[79] however, did not find a difference in survival between metabolic responders and nonresponders, although there was a trend toward improved survival in patients who demonstrated a lower post-gefitinib SUV of less than 7 at 2 days. These studies confirm that an early metabolic response on PET, in the absence of tumor shrinkage, can provide a clinically meaningful assessment of therapeutic activity in NSCLC.

Nevertheless, it is difficult to ascertain the optimal timing of scans after commencement of treatment because a reduction in tumor size in lung cancer can take time. Furthermore, molecular targeted therapies have been shown to work via inhibiting cell growth (cytostasis) and in some cases may not cause tumor regression but rather decrease tumor growth rate, resulting in prolonged stable disease. Similarly, immune therapeutic agents used in lung cancer enhance antitumor immune response, resulting in durable stable disease, which may be viewed as an indicator of meaningful therapeutic effect. Besides, inflammatory reaction and fibrosis formation can increase FDG uptake, confounding the assessment of tumor response early on.[76] Timing of response assessment depends on the type of therapy the patient is receiving, and although there are currently no approved guidelines, tumor response assessment is usually performed at baseline and after several weeks or months of therapy (between 6 weeks and 3 months).

PET DETECTION OF OLIGOPROGRESSIVE DISEASE

The most common utility of PET in the clinical setting thus far is in detecting oligometastatic disease, which occurs early in the metastatic process defined by a small number of new metastases with limited progression of disease. It is also useful in determining the best site to biopsy, especially in cases where tumor recurrence is uncertain. Increasingly, patients with *EGFR* mutation-positive and *ALK* rearranged NSCLC with oligoprogressive disease are being treated with a combination of local therapy (surgery, standard radiotherapy, or stereotactic radiotherapy) and continuation of systemic therapy, which appears to translate into improved outcomes.[80] Therefore, the early identification of oligoprogressive disease on PET is valuable to enable a change in treatment decision.

SUMMARY

In the last few years, substantial progress has been made in the discovery of genomic alterations of lung cancer, illuminating clinically significant somatic mutations and enabling further refinement in the subclassification of NSCLC. The identification of oncogenic drivers together with molecular targeted therapies and newer immunotherapies have changed the way patients with lung cancer are treated, with considerable progress still to be made therapeutically. Functional imaging with PET can provide an early indication of therapeutic response in patients receiving cytostatic agents, including predicting disease recurrence in patients receiving curative intent treatment. As newer therapies emerge in NSCLC, more advanced imaging modality and novel PET tracers will be required as pharmacodynamic measures of therapy efficacy, along with early predictors of treatment response.

REFERENCES

1. Molina JR, Ying P, Cassivi SD, et al. Non-small cell lung cancer: epidemiology, risk factors, treatment and survivorship. Mayo Clin Proc 2008;83:584–94.
2. Hicks RJ. Role of 18F-FDG PET in assessment of response in non-small cell lung cancer. J Nucl Med 2009;50:31S–42S.
3. Ding L, Getz G, Wheeler DA, et al. Somatic mutations affect key pathways in lung adenocarcinoma. Nature 2008;455(7216):1069–75.
4. Swanton C, Govindan R. Clinical implications of genomic discoveries in lung cancer. N Engl J Med 2016;374(19):1864–73.
5. Cancer Genome Atlas Research Network. Comprehensive molecular profiling of lung adenocarcinoma. Nature 2014;511(7511):543–50.
6. Larsen JE, Minna JD. Molecular biology of lung cancer: clinical implications. Clin Chest Med 2011;32(4):703–40.
7. Kris MG, Johnson BE, Berry LD, et al. Using multiplexed assays of oncogenic drivers in lung cancers to select targeted drugs. JAMA 2014;311:1998–2006.
8. Weinstein IB, Joe A. Oncogene addiction. Cancer Res 2008;68(9):3077–80 [discussion: 3080].
9. Levy MA, Lovly CM, Pao W. Translating genomic information into clinical medicine: lung cancer as a paradigm. Genome Res 2012;22(11):2101–8.
10. Barlesi F, Mazieres J, Merlio JP, et al. Routine molecular profiling of patients with advanced non-small-cell lung cancer: results of a 1 year nationwide programme of the French cooperative thoracic intergroup (IFCT). Lancet Oncol 2016;387:1–12.
11. Cancer Genome Atlas Research Network. Comprehensive genomic characterization of squamous cell lung cancers. Nature 2012;489(7417):519–25.
12. Haura EB, Tanvetyanon T, Chiappori A, et al. Phase I/II study of the Src inhibitor dasatinib in combination with erlotinib in advanced non-small-cell lung cancer. J Clin Oncol 2010;28(8):1387–94.
13. Johnson FM, Bekele BN, Feng L, et al. Phase II study of dasatinib in patients with advanced non-small-cell lung cancer. J Clin Oncol 2010;28(30):4609–15.
14. Desai A, Adjei AA. FGFR signalling as a target for lung cancer therapy. J Thorac Oncol 2015;11:9–20.
15. Mac Manus MP, Hicks RJ, Matthews JP, et al. Positron emission tomography is superior to computed tomography scanning for response-assesment after radical radiotherapy or chemoradiotherapy in patients with non-small cell lung cancer. J Clin Oncol 2003;21:1285–92.
16. Lardinois D, Weder W, Hany TF, et al. Staging of non-small-cell lung cancer with integrated positron-emission tomography and computed tomography. N Engl J Med 2003;348(25):2500–7.
17. Jadvar H, Alavi A, Gambhir SS. 18F-FDG uptake in lung, breast, and colon cancers: molecular biology correlates and disease characterization. J Nucl Med 2009;50(11):1820–7.
18. Fischer B, Lassen U, Mortensen J, et al. Preoperative staging of lung cancer with combined PET-CT. N Engl J Med 2011;361:32–9.
19. Lindeman NI, Cagle PT, Beasley B, et al. Molecular testing guideline for selection of lung cancer patients for EGFR and ALK tyrosine kinase inhibitors. Arch Pathol Lab Med 2013;137:828–60.
20. Sequist LV, Soria JC, Goldman JW, et al. Rociletinib in EGFR-mutated non-small cell lung cancer. N Engl J Med 2015;372:1700–9.
21. Mok TS, Wu Y-L, Thongprasert S, et al. Gefitinib or carboplatin-paclitaxel in pulmonary adenocarcinoma. N Engl J Med 2009;361:947–57.
22. Inoue A, Kobayashi K, Maemondo M, et al. Updated overall survival results from a randomized phase III trial comparing gefitinib with carboplatin-paclitaxel for chemo-naive non-small cell lung cancer with sensitive EGFR gene mutations (NEJ002). Ann Oncol 2013;24:54–9.
23. Mitsudomi T, Morita S, Yatabe Y, et al. Gefitinib versus cisplatin plus docetaxel in patients with non-small-cell lung cancer harbouring mutations of the epidermal growth factor receptor (WJTOG3405): an open label, randomised phase 3 trial. Lancet Oncol 2010;11:121–8.
24. Rosell R, Carcereny C, Gervais R, et al. Erlotinib versus standard chemotherapy as first-line treatment for European patients with advanced EGFR mutation-positive non-small cell lung cancer (EURTAC): a multicentre, open-label, randomised phase 3 trial. Lancet Oncol 2012;13:239–46.
25. Sequist LV, Yang J, Yamamoto N, et al. Phase III study of afatinib or cisplatin plus pemetrexed in patients with metastatic lung adenocarcinoma with EGFR mutations. J Clin Oncol 2013;31:3327–34.
26. Wu YL, Zhou C, Hu CP, et al. Afatinib versus cisplatin plus gemcitabine for first-line treatment of Asian patients with advanced non-small-cell lung cancer harbouring EGFR mutations (LUX-Lung 6): an open-label, randomised phase 3 trial. Lancet Oncol 2014;15:213–22.
27. Zhou C, Wu YL, Chen G, et al. Erlotinib versus chemotherapy as first-line treatment for patients with advanced EGFR mutation-positive non-small-cell lung cancer (OPTIMAL, CTONG-0802): a multicentre, open-label, randomized, phase 3 study. Lancet Oncol 2011;12:735–42.
28. Yang J, Wu Y-L, Schuler M, et al. Afatinib versus cisplatin-based chemotherapy for EGFR

mutation-positive lung adenocarcinoma (LUX-Lung 3 and LUX-Lung 6): analysis of overall survival data from two randomised, phase 3 trials. Lancet Oncol 2015;16:141–51.

29. Solomon B, Varella-Garcia M, Camidge DR. ALK gene rearrangements a new therapeutic target in a molecularly defined subset of non-small cell lung cancer. J Thorac Oncol 2009;4:1450–4.

30. Cameron L, Solomon B. New treatment options for ALK-rearranged non-small cell lung cancer. Curr Treat Options Oncol 2015;16:1–14.

31. Solomon B, Mok T, Kim D-W, et al. First-line crizotinib versus chemotherapy in ALK-positive lung cancer. N Engl J Med 2015;371:2167–77.

32. Soria JC, Tan DS, Chiari R, et al. First-line ceritinib versus platinum-based chemotherapy in advanced ALK-rearranged non-small-cell lung cancer (ASCEND-4): a randomised, open-label, phase 3 study. Lancet 2017;389(10072):917–29.

33. Sprouffske K, Merlo LM, Gerrish PJ, et al. Cancer in light of experimental evolution. Curr Biol 2012;22(17):R762–71.

34. Fisher R, Pusztai L, Swanton C. Cancer heterogeneity: implications for targeted therapeutics. Br J Cancer 2013;108:479–85.

35. Jamal-Hanjani M, Hackshaw A, Ngai Y, et al. Tracking genomic cancer evolution for precision medicine: the lung TRACERx study. PLoS Biol 2014;12(7):e1001906.

36. Gerlinger M, Rowan AJ, Horswell S, et al. Intratumor heterogeneity and branched evolution revealed by multiregion sequencing. N Engl J Med 2012;366(10):883–92.

37. Engleman JA, Jänne PA. Mechanisms of acquired resistance to epidermal growth factor receptor tyrosine kinase inhibitors in non-small cell lung cancer. Clin Cancer Res 2008;14:2895–9.

38. Janne PA, Yang JC-Y, Kim DW, et al. AZD9291 in EGFR inhibitor-resistant non-small cell lung cancer. N Engl J Med 2015;372:1689–99.

39. Karlovich CGJ, Sun J-M, Mann E, et al. Assessment of EGFR mutation status in matched plasma and tumour tissue of NSCLC patients from a phase 1 study of rociletinib (CO-1686). Clin Cancer Res 2016;22(10):2386–95.

40. Piotrowska ZNM, Karlovich CA, Wakelee HA, et al. Heterogeneity underlies the emergence of EGFR T790M wild-type clones following treatment of T790M-positive cancers with a third generation EGFR inhibitor. Cancer Discov 2015;5(7):713–22.

41. Watanabe MKT, Isa S, Ando M, et al. Ultra-sensitive detection of pretreatment EGFR T790M mutation in non-small cell lung cancer patients with an EGFR-activating mutation using droplet digital PCR. Clin Cancer Res 2015;21(15):3552–60.

42. Daniel CB, Kobayashi SS. Whacking a mole-cule: clinical activity and mechanisms of resistance to third generation EGFR inhibitors in EGFR mutated lung cancers with EGFR-T790M. Transl Lung Cancer Res 2015;4(6):809–15.

43. Cross DAS, Ghiorghiu S, Eberlein C, et al. AZD9291, an irreversible EGFR TKI, overcomes T790M-mediated resistance to EGFR inhibitors in lung cancer. Cancer Discov 2014;4:9.

44. Mok TS, Wu YL, Ahn MJ, et al. Osimertinib or platinum-pemetrexed in EGFR T790M-positive lung cancer. N Engl J Med 2017;376(7):629–40.

45. Thress KS, Paweletz CP, Felip E, et al. Acquired EGFR C797S mutation mediates resistance to AZD9291 in non-small cell lung cancer harboring EGFR T790M. Nat Med 2015;21:1–5.

46. Gainor JF, Dardaei L, Yoda S, et al. Molecular mechanisms of resistance to first- and second-generation ALK inhibitors in ALK-rearranged lung Cancer. Cancer Discov 2016;6(10):1118–33.

47. Tiseo M, Ippolito M, Scarlattei M, et al. Predictive and prognostic value of early response assessment using 18FDG-PET in advanced non-small cell lung cancer patients treated with erlotinib. Cancer Chemother Pharmacol 2014;73(2):299–307.

48. Wahl RL, Jacene H, Kasamon Y, et al. From RECIST to PERCIST: evolving considerations for PET. J Nucl Med 2009;50:122S–50S.

49. Blumenthal GM, Karuri SW, Zhang H, et al. Overall response rate, progression-free survival, and overall survival with targeted and standard therapies in advanced non-small-cell lung cancer: US Food and Drug Administration trial-level and patient-level analyses. J Clin Oncol 2015;33(9):1008–14.

50. Wolchok JD, Hoos A, O'Day S, et al. Guidelines for the evaluation of immune therapy activity in solid tumors: immune-related response criteria. Clin Cancer Res 2009;15(23):7412–20.

51. Nishino M, Hatabu H, Johnson BE, et al. State of the art: response assessment in lung cancer in the era of genomic medicine. Radiology 2014;271(1):6–27.

52. Young H, Baum R, Cremerius U, et al. Measurement of clinical and subclinical tumour response using [18F]-fluorodeoxyglucose and positron emission tomography: review and 1999 EORTC recommendations. Eur J Cancer 1999;35:1773–82.

53. Reck M, Rodriguez-Abreu D, Robinson AG, et al. Pembrolizumab versus chemotherapy for PD-L1-positive non-small-cell lung cancer. N Engl J Med 2016;375(19):1823–33.

54. Brahmer J, Reckamp KL, Baas P, et al. Nivolumab versus docetaxel in advanced squamous-cell non-small-cell lung cancer. N Engl J Med 2015;373(2):123–35.

55. Borghaei H, Paz-Ares L, Horn L, et al. Nivolumab versus docetaxel in advanced nonsquamous non-small-cell lung cancer. N Engl J Med 2015;373(17):1627–39.

56. Duhaylongsod F, Lowe VJ, Patz EF, et al. Lung tumour growth correlates with glucose metabolism measured by fluoride-18 fluorodeoxyglucose positron emission tomography. Ann Thorac Surg 1995; 60:1348–52.

57. Su H, Bodenstein C, Dumont RA, et al. Monitoring tumor glucose utilization by positron emission tomography for the prediction of treatment response to epidermal growth factor receptor kinase inhibitors. Clin Cancer Res 2006;12(19):5659–67.

58. Nguyen XC, Lee WW, Chung JH, et al. FDG uptake, glucose transporter type 1, and Ki-67 expressions in non-small-cell lung cancer: correlations and prognostic values. Eur J Radiol 2007;62(2):214–9.

59. Mak RH, Digumarthy SR, Muzikansky A, et al. Role of 18F-fluorodeoxyglucose positron emission tomography in predicting epidermal growth factor receptor mutations in non-small cell lung cancer. Oncologist 2011;16(3):319–26.

60. Brown RS, Leung JY, Kison PV, et al. Glucose transporters and FDG uptake in untreated primary human non-small cell lung cancer. J Nucl Med 1999;40: 556–65.

61. Simons AL, Orcutt KP, Madsen JM, et al. The role of AKT pathway signaling in glocuse metabolism and metabolic oxidative stress. In: Oxidative Stress in Cancer Biology and Therapy. Springer Science & Business Media: New York; 2012. p. 22–35.

62. Mileshkin L, Hicks RJ, Hughes BG, et al. Changes in FDG- and FLT-PET imaging in patients with non-small cell lung cancer treated with erlotinib. Clin Cancer Res 2011;17:3304–15.

63. Kubota R, Yamada S, Kubota K, et al. Intratumoral distribution of fluorine-18-fluorodeoxyglucose in vivo: high accumulation in macrophages and granulation tissues studied by microautoradiography. J Nucl Med 1992;33(11):1972–80.

64. Shields AF, Grierson JR, Dohmen BM, et al. Imaging proliferation in vivo with [F-18]FLT and positron emission tomography. Nat Med 1998;4(11):1334–6.

65. Barthel H, Cleij MC, Collingridge DR, et al. 3 -Deoxy-3-[18F]fluorothymidine as a new marker for monitoring tumor response to antiproliferative therapy in vivo with positron emission tomography. Cancer Res 2003;63:3791–8.

66. Ullrich RT, Zander T, Neumaier B, et al. Early detection of erlotinib treatment response in NSCLC by 3'-deoxy-3'-[F]-fluoro-L-thymidine ([F]FLT) positron emission tomography (PET). PLoS One 2008;3(12):e3908.

67. Buck AK, Schirrmeister H, Hetzel M, et al. 3-Deoxy-3-[18F]fluorothymidine-positron emission tomography for noninvasive assessment of proliferation in pulmonary nodules. Cancer Res 2002;62:3331–4.

68. Bahce I, Yaqub M, Smit EF, et al. Personalizing NSCLC therapy by characterizing tumors using TKI-PET and immuno-PET. Lung Cancer 2017;107: 1–13.

69. Memon AA, Jakobsen S, Dagnaes-Hansen F, et al. Positron emission tomography (PET) imaging with [11C]-labeled erlotinib: a micro-PET study on mice with lung tumor xenografts. Cancer Res 2009; 69(3):873–8.

70. Memon AA, Weber B, Winterdahl M, et al. PET imaging of patients with non-small cell lung cancer employing an EGF receptor targeting drug as tracer. Br J Cancer 2011;105(12):1850–5.

71. Rittmeyer A, Barlesi F, Waterkamp D, et al. Atezolizumab versus docetaxel in patients with previously treated non-small-cell lung cancer (OAK): a phase 3, open-label, multicentre randomised controlled trial. Lancet 2017;389(10066):255–65.

72. Bensch F, van der Veen E, Jorritsma A, et al. First-in-human PET imaging with the PD-L1 antibody 89-Zr-atezolizumab. AACR Washington, DC, April 1–5, 2017.

73. Stroobants S, Goeminne J, Seegers M, et al. 18FDG-positron emission tomography for the early prediction of response in advanced soft tissue sarcoma treated with imatinib mesylate (Glivec). Eur J Cancer 2003;39(14):2012–20.

74. Sunaga N, Oriuchi N, Kaira K, et al. Usefulness of FDG-PET for early prediction of the response to gefitinib in non-small cell lung cancer. Lung Cancer 2008;59(2):203–10.

75. Sohn HJ, Yang YJ, Ryu JS, et al. [18F]Fluorothymidine positron emission tomography before and 7 days after gefitinib treatment predicts response in patients with advanced adenocarcinoma of the lung. Clin Cancer Res 2008;14(22):7423–9.

76. van Gool MH, Aukema TS, Hartemink KJ, et al. FDG-PET/CT response evaluation during EGFR-TKI treatment in patients with NSCLC. World J Radiol 2014;6: 392–8.

77. Zander T, Scheffler M, Nogova L, et al. Early prediction of nonprogression in advanced non-small-cell lung cancer treated with erlotinib by using [(18)F]fluorodeoxyglucose and [(18)F]fluorothymidine positron emission tomography. J Clin Oncol 2011; 29(13):1701–8.

78. Soto Parra H, Ippolito M, Tiseo, M, et al. Usefulness of 18FDG-positron emission tomography (FDG-PET) for early prediction of erlotinib (Eb) treatment outcome in non-small cell lung cancer (NSCLC) patients: results of a pilot study. 2009;27. [Abstract 7568].

79. Takahashi R, Hirata H, Tachibana I, et al. Early [18F] fuorodeoxyglucose positron emission tomography at two days of gefitinib treatment predicts clinical outcome in patients with adenocarcinoma of the lung. Clin Cancer Res 2012;18:220–8.

80. Weickhardt AJ, Scheier B, Burke JM, et al. Local ablative therapy of oligoprogressive disease prolongs disease control by tyrosine kinase inhibitors in oncogene-addicted non-small-cell lung cancer. J Thorac Oncol 2012;7(12):1807–14.

Treatment Planning for Radiation Therapy

Michael MacManus, MD, FRANZCR[a,b,*], Sarah Everitt, PhD[a,b]

KEYWORDS

- Lung cancer • PET • CT scanning • Radiation therapy • Surgery • Chemotherapy

KEY POINTS

- ^{18}F-fluorodeoxyglucose (FDG)–PET scanning is an essential part of the pretreatment evaluation for patients with lung cancer who are candidates for curative-intent radiation therapy.
- PET data are critical to the radiation treatment planning process and contemporary images acquired on a combined PET/computed tomography scanner in the radiotherapy treatment position are the ideal images for target volume delineation in patients with locoregionally advanced disease.
- Response-adapted therapy, based on PET images acquired during the treatment course, is a promising experimental approach.
- Although metabolic tumor imaging with FDG remains the standard approach, imaging of proliferation and hypoxia with alternative tracers may give additional information.
- Uptake of FDG in irradiated normal tissues may have application in the diagnosis and management of radiation-induced toxicity.

INTRODUCTION

Treatment planning for patients with lung cancer who are candidates for potentially curative radiation therapy (RT) is a broad topic that encompasses many factors, including staging, selection of appropriate patients, and target volume definition. In all of these critical areas, imaging plays a central role.[1] Although ^{18}F-fluorodeoxyglucose (FDG)–PET imaging is currently the most important modality for staging disease extent and for defining the target volume for patients with lung cancer who are treated with RT,[2] many other factors should be considered important when deciding between surgery or an attempt at potentially curative RT or a less aggressive palliative treatment regimen. As stereotactic ablative RT (SABR)[3] has become more widely used for potentially curative treatment of small lung tumors and oligometastases (Fig. 1), the interface between surgery and RT has become more complex and controversial.

With advances in the systemic treatment of lung cancer, such as targeted therapies including epidermal growth factor receptor (EGFR) tyrosine kinase inhibitors (TKIs),[4] novel indications for RT are being pioneered. For example, after a good initial treatment response to TKI, patients with oligoprogressive disease may respond to local RT and continue to benefit from their systemic therapy at other disease sites that remain controlled (Fig. 2). Accurate imaging is important in such cases to ensure that disease progression is truly localized. As treatment paradigms become more complex, the integration of imaging into the overall management of the patient becomes more subtle and refined. This

Disclosures: Neither author has any relevant disclosures.
[a] Department of Radiation Oncology, Division of Radiation Oncology and Cancer Imaging, Peter MacCallum Cancer Centre, 305 Grattan Street, Melbourne, Victoria 3000, Australia; [b] The Sir Peter MacCallum Department of Oncology, The University of Melbourne, Parkville, Victoria 3010, Australia
* Corresponding author. Department of Radiation Oncology, Peter MacCallum Cancer Centre, 305 Grattan Street, Melbourne, Victoria 3000, Australia.
E-mail address: michael.macmanus@petermac.org

PET Clin 13 (2018) 43–57
http://dx.doi.org/10.1016/j.cpet.2017.08.005
1556-8598/18/© 2017 Elsevier Inc. All rights reserved.

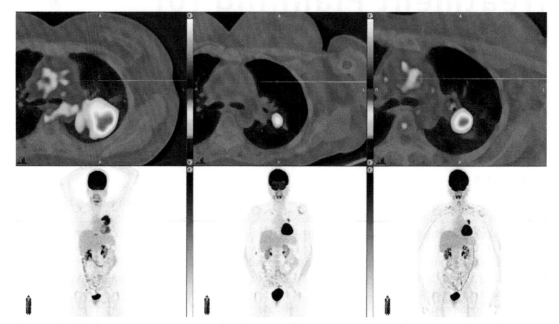

Fig. 1. Role of radiation in a patient treated with targeted therapy. Sequential FDG-PET/computed tomography (CT) (*top row*) and PET (*bottom row*) images for a patient with stage epidermal growth factor receptor (EGFR) mutation–positive stage IV NSCLC. On the 2 left images, a painful metastasis at T9 and the left lower lobe primary tumor can be observed. The 2 middle images, performed 19 months later, after local irradiation at T9 and with ongoing anti-EGFR tyrosine kinase inhibitor (TKI) therapy, show an ongoing complete response at the site of irradiation and an excellent partial response in the primary tumor. After a further 3 months (2 right images), there is continuing disease control at the irradiated site but progression in the primary tumor.

article focuses on non–small cell lung cancer (NSCLC) rather than small cell lung cancer (SCLC) because the literature is much larger and more conclusive for this group of diseases, although the role of FDG-PET scanning in SCLC is becoming better established because of the high incremental value of PET imaging in this more aggressive but less common cancer.

WHAT PATIENTS ARE SUITABLE FOR CURATIVE-INTENT RADIATION THERAPY?
Disease-Related Factors

In general, patients who have NSCLC that can be resected without a high risk of death or severe morbidity are recommended to have surgery. Curative surgery generally involves a lobectomy or pneumonectomy and mediastinal lymph node dissection but in selected small T1 tumors a more limited sublobar resection may be considered. Stage I and II patients may not be fit for surgery because of comorbidities such as lung or heart disease but may still be eligible for curative-intent RT. Selected patients with T1 and T2 tumors that are located 2 cm or more beyond the major airways may be suitable for SABR, in

which an extremely high ablative RT dose is delivered by multiple narrow noncoplanar beams in a small number of very-high-dose fractions (or a single fraction). In appropriately selected patients, local disease control is very high (around 90%) after SABR and survival may be comparable with surgery. More centrally located T1 tumors are more safely treated with conventionally fractionated RT.

In contrast with earlier stage disease, most patients with stage III NSCLC are better served by radical concurrent platinum-based chemoradiation with curative intent rather than by surgery, and for these patients long-term survival rates have increased incrementally in recent years, in large part because of the use of PET for patient selection. In the special case of limited stage IIIA disease with single nodal station and potentially resectable N2 disease there is continuing controversy around the use of surgery after neoadjuvant therapy with induction chemotherapy or after induction chemoradiation. Trimodality therapy may provide superior local disease control for patients who have stage IIIA disease amenable to resection by lobectomy. However, it is not clear that overall survival is improved compared with chemoradiation alone.

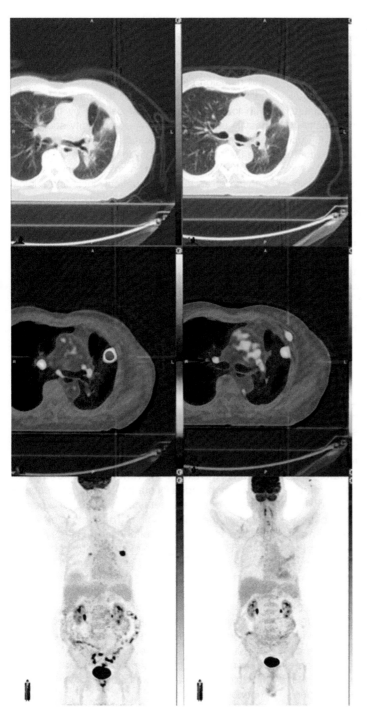

Fig. 2. Baseline (*left column*) and 2 months after treatment (*right column*) FDG-PET/CT scans of a patient treated with SABR (26 Gy in a single fraction) for recurrent NSCLC. Rows from top to bottom show CT, fused PET/CT, and PET views respectively. Despite the presence of a persistent mass on the posttreatment CT image (*right upper panel*) the PET images show low FDG uptake consistent with a complete metabolic response.

Patients who are suitable for treatment with curative-intent RT must have disease that can be encompassed within a tolerable RT target volume. In patients with large tumors or with multiple sites of nodal involvement, suitability for RT may only be definitively determined if a radiation treatment plan is created and normal tissue constraints can be met. In borderline cases, the patient may accept a very high risk of complications in an effort to control the cancer or a lower dose of radiation may be prescribed in order to meet a predefined set of normal tissue constraints. This isotoxic approach delivers the highest dose that is considered acceptably safe. Because there is no standard curative dose of radiation, doses less than the widely used 60 Gy or an equivalent schedule may still be enough to cure some patients with radiosensitive tumors. A very small proportion of patients can be cured with lower palliative doses of radiation. The use of a higher RT dose in radical chemoradiation was not found to be associated with superior survival but caused more toxicity in the landmark Radiation Therapy Oncology Group (RTOG) 0617 randomized controlled trial of 60 versus 74 Gy.[5,6]

The increasing use of PET has helped to identify patients with oligometastatic disease, especially single sites of extracranial metastasis. The superior survival associated with single extracranial metastases has been recognized in the recent eighth edition of the staging manual.[7] They may undergo surgery or curative-intent RT to the thorax and SABR[8,9] or surgery to the solitary metastasis. It is not yet clear what proportion of patients with synchronous solitary intrathoracic M1a or extrathoracic M1b disease treated with aggressive therapy to all disease sites may be cured, and further studies are required.

Patient Factors

If a patient is not suitable for surgery but is potentially curable with RT, patient factors other than disease extent must be also considered before deciding on treatment. These factors include global factors such as performance status and weight loss and the function of specific organs, especially the lungs and the heart. One of the most important patient-related factors is performance status. Patients with lung cancer with an Eastern Cooperative Oncology Group (ECOG) performance status of 2 or worse have a poor prognosis. In such cases, nonaggressive palliative approaches are usually more appropriate. Aggressive treatment may still be considered if poor performance status onset has been rapid and is potentially responsive to therapy such as superior vena-caval obstruction or rapid occlusion of a major airway. Weight loss of greater than 10% body mass is also a negative prognostic factor and is often associated with advanced disease and/or severe emphysema.

NSCLC is overwhelmingly a disease caused by tobacco consumption and patients with NSCLC often have other diseases related to smoking, including emphysema and ischemic heart disease. It is increasingly common for a new lung cancer to arise in a patient who has been successfully treated for a previous lung or head and neck cancer. The effects of previous resections or RT must be considered when planning a new course of

curative treatment in these cases. It is important to document the physiologic factors that will affect the patient's ability to safely undergo therapy. Respiratory function tests, including spirometry and diffusion capacity for carbon monoxide, can help estimate the ability of the patient to cope with loss of lung function caused by fibrosis of heavily irradiated lung. A comorbidity score may be used to help select suitable patients for aggressive therapies.[10,11] Ideally in NSCLC all of the factors that are important in making the treatment choice for an individual patient, including clinical and physiologic factors, pathology, and imaging studies, should be discussed at a multidisciplinary meeting and a comprehensive management plan agreed.

USE OF IMAGING IN STAGING AND SELECTING PATIENTS FOR CURATIVE-INTENT RADIATION THERAPY

Accurate staging of lung cancer ensures that patients selected for RT have potentially curable disease. The results of a range of different investigations, including bronchoscopy, mediastinoscopy (if performed), biopsies, and imaging studies are integrated to determine the final stage grouping. Patients with locoregionally advanced disease do not typically undergo extensive surgical staging and knowledge of the true extent of the primary tumor and its potential resectability (T stage), the extent of involvement of the intrathoracic lymph nodes (N stage), and the presence or absence of distant metastases (M stage) is gained primarily through imaging. The increasing availability of endoscopic bronchoscopic ultrasonography (EBUS)–guided[12] biopsy has helped further increase the accuracy of assessment of intrathoracic disease status and guide RT planning.

Although computed tomography (CT) scanning has long been the workhorse of lung cancer imaging it has significant weaknesses that require the addition of other imaging modalities. For example, combined CT and magnetic resonance (MR) imaging can help to characterize the extent of extrathoracic soft tissue extension in patients with superior sulcus tumors.[13]

However, the advent of FDG-PET scanning exposed significant limitations of structural imaging in lung cancer staging, including the poor performance of CT in correctly assessing intrathoracic lymph node status and in detecting extracranial distant metastasis. The use of FDG-PET has globally increased the accuracy of lung cancer staging, especially when patients with more advanced tumors are candidates for RT. The lower resolution of PET is more than compensated for by its high tumor to normal tissue contrast. The fusion of PET and CT data to produce hybrid PET/CT images allows the strengths of both modalities to complement one another and to compensate for each other's weaknesses. The resulting fused images are by far the best currently available starting point for the use of imaging to stage lung cancer and to define target volumes for RT.

Mediastinal Nodal Staging

CT-based estimation of lymph node status in NSCLC depends entirely on nodal dimensions.[14] Lymph nodes with short-axis transverse diameters greater than 1 cm are considered to be positive. Textural analysis may increase the accuracy of lymph node assessment with CT.[15] However, tumor is often present in smaller nodes and large nodes may be reactive or enlarged because of inflammatory or infective disease. Changing the cutoff diameter for assignment of nodal status in either direction simply increases the false-positive or false-negative rate.

FDG-PET has dramatically enhanced the ability to correctly classify the status of intrathoracic lymph nodes. Mediastinal staging paradigms that include PET, especially when both PET and CT are considered, are dramatically more accurate than CT alone. In the Gould[16] meta-analysis, FDG-PET was much more accurate than CT for lymph node classification ($P<.001$). Median sensitivity and specificity were only 61% and 79% respectively for CT but, for PET, sensitivity and specificity were 85% and 90% respectively. When CT showed enlarged lymph nodes, PET was more sensitive but less specific (median sensitivity, 100%; median specificity, 78%) when CT showed normal-sized nodes (sensitivity, 82%; specificity, 93%; $P = .002$). The most accurate approach for intrathoracic nodal staging uses combined PET/CT images and this is more cost-effective than no-PET approaches.[17] Despite its high level of accuracy, PET/CT is not perfect and the selective use of nodal biopsy with mediastinoscopy[18] or with EBUS[12,19] can be helpful in selected cases for determining which nodal stations need to be included in RT target volumes.

Determination of Local Tumor Extent

Lung tumors surrounded by healthy lung are usually well visualized by CT. However, when tumors invade or contact intrathoracic structures that have similar CT density to themselves, such as mediastinal or apical soft tissues or atelectatic lung, tumor margins may not be visible and CT becomes unreliable for defining local tumor extent

and designing radiation target volumes. Making the volume big enough to cover all possible tumor extensions would unnecessarily irradiate large volumes of non–tumor-bearing normal tissues in many cases.

FDG-PET can usually distinguish between atelectatic lung[20,21] and the underlying tumor that has caused the lobe or lung to collapse. This ability has the potential to greatly increase the accuracy of RT planning in such cases, avoiding geographic miss and preventing unnecessary lung irradiation (**Fig. 3**). Similarly, with apical lung tumors, PET/CT may reveal previously unsuspected extrathoracic tumor extension and more accurately portray invasion of the mediastinum, vertebral bodies, and intervertebral foramina. In some settings, MR imaging provides additional complementary information to PET/CT.

Patients with locally advanced lung cancers often have additional nodules in nearby lung tissue, which could represent satellite nodules, nodal metastases, or blood-borne metastases. Nodules without FDG uptake are unlikely to be malignant, unless they are too small to characterize, but FDG-avid pulmonary lesions are likely to be malignant in patients with lung cancer[22] if there is no other plausible explanation, such as tuberculosis or fungal infection. It is rarely possible to biopsy all such lesions and a pragmatic decision is generally taken to include them in the RT target volume if the irradiated volume will not be too large. PET may also show the presence of pleural metastases that are not visible or appear as nonspecific pleural thickening on CT scans. This finding usually precludes a curative-intent treatment course.

Patients who present with solitary pulmonary nodules[22] often have chronic lung disease, often tobacco related, such as emphysema with large bullae, which can make biopsy hazardous. In patients in whom lung disease precludes both a safe attempt at needle biopsy and a curative surgical resection, the demonstration of high FDG uptake on PET and the characteristic CT appearance of lung cancer can be regarded as sufficient evidence to allow the patient to proceed to curative-intent treatment with SABR or conventional RT.[23]

Detection of Distant Metastasis

Routine CT scanning of the chest and upper abdomen is insufficient to screen for distant metastasis in patients with NSCLC who are being considered for curative-intent treatment, especially those with locoregionally advanced tumors. For staging of the brain, MR imaging is clearly superior to CT and both CT and MR imaging are

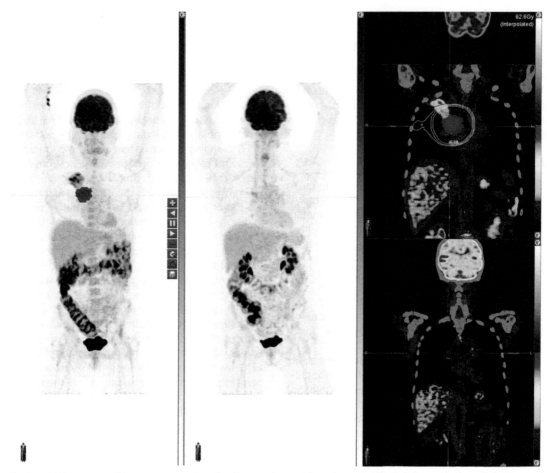

Fig. 3. PET/CT scan used for treatment planning in a patient with atelectasis. The left 2 panels show baseline and postchemoradiation (60 Gy) FDG-PET scans for a patient with NSCLC associated with atelectasis of the right upper lobe. In the baseline panel, the radiation-planning isodoses are superimposed, showing that much of the atelectatic lung has been spared. The right upper panel shows a coronal fused PET/CT image of the baseline scan, also with the isodose lines superimposed. The lower right hand panel shows a coronal fused PET/CT image of the post-treatment scan, showing a complete metabolic response to therapy and resolution of atelectasis.

more sensitive than FDG-PET for the detection of small brain metastases because of the high normal background uptake of FDG in the brain.[24,25] However, the addition of FDG-PET to the staging process greatly increases the probability that extracranial distant metastasis will be detected. Because acquisition of whole-body PET/CT images is routine, and because of the high uptake of FDG in metastases in lung cancer, the additional yield from PET in detecting unsuspected extracranial sites of metastasis is high.[26]

Although overall staging efficiency is increased, the incremental value of PET is most apparent at several critical anatomic sites. The adrenal gland is a common site of metastasis in lung cancer but benign adrenal enlargement is fairly common. FDG-PET imaging both increases the accuracy of assessment of adrenal enlargement[27] and can

often detect metastasis in nonenlarged adrenals. Similarly, for the detection of bone metastasis,[28] PET can often detect osseous metastasis at sites that appear normal on CT, have nonspecific CT abnormalities, or are outside the field of view of the CT scan. Radionuclide bone scanning also routinely images the whole body but it is much less specific and accurate than PET. Liver metastases often have CT density comparable with normal liver and are commonly seen on PET scans when they are not apparent on CT.[29]

In NSCLC, the probability that PET will detect unsuspected metastasis increases with the extent of disease apparent on pre-PET imaging, consistent with the Bayes theorem. In one prospective study, a group of 167 patients with pre-PET stage I to III NSCLC underwent staging FDG-PET scans. The probability that PET would detect distant metastasis increased with the pre-PET stage from I (7.5%) through II (18%) to III (24%, $P = .016$). The risk of PET-detected metastasis was significantly higher in stage III compared with stages I to II ($P = .039$).[26] Although FDG-PET is insensitive for the detection of intracranial metastasis, other PET tracers can overcome this limitation. The proliferation tracer ^{18}F-fluorothymidine (FLT), which has low cerebral uptake, detected brain metastases in 3 of 60 patients who were prospectively imaged with FLT-PET.[30]

Impact of ^{18}F-fluorodeoxyglucose–PET on overall management strategy of patients with non–small cell lung cancer with radiation therapy

Soon after PET was adopted for staging and selecting patients for curative-intent RT, it became clear that overall survival (OS) would be superior compared with non–PET-staged cohorts managed similarly, in large part because of the exclusion of incurable patients with PET-detected advanced disease from futile curative-intent RT or chemoRT. In a study that compared early survival in 80 PET-staged and 77 non–PET-staged patients treated with radical RT, mortality in the first year was 17% and 8% for PET patients and 32% and 4% for non-PET patients, respectively.[31] The hazard ratio for NSCLC mortality for PET versus non-PET patients was 0.55 ($P = .0075$) after adjusting for differences in the use of concurrent chemotherapy, which significantly improved survival.

When stand-alone PET was used prospectively to stage 153 candidates for curative-intent RT, the 46 patients (30%) who received palliative therapies after PET because of PET-detected advanced disease had much worse OS ($P = .02$), consistent with appropriate PET-based decision making.[21] When PET/CT was used in a similar Australian prospective study, only 66% of patients were selected for curative therapy. OS for patients treated with curative intent was 77.5% and 35.6% at 1 and 4 years, respectively. OS for palliatively treated patients was only 16.3% and 4.1% at 1 and 4 years, respectively ($P<.001$).[32] In these series PET not only directed changes from curative to palliative treatments but also appropriately changed treatment from RT to surgery in a small proportion of cases with false-positive nodes on CT. A similar impact of PET has been reported by a study from Poland,[33] in which only 75 of 100 patients intended for radical RT received it and, in those cases in which RT was delivered, 27% of patients would have experienced geographic miss of gross tumor without PET.

Timeliness of treatment-planning PET/computed tomography scans

Locoregionally advanced lung cancers can progress rapidly in the interval between initial staging and the commencement of RT.[34] Everitt and colleagues[35] investigated tumor progression that occurred between staging and RT-planning FDG-PET/CT scans in 28 NSCLC patients. The median interval between scans was 24 days and tumor, node, metastasis (TNM) stage progression was detected in 11 patients (39%). The risk of being upstaged within 24 days was 32%. In 8 patients (29%), treatment was changed to palliation. Patients with progression between staging and RT-planning PET scans have a grave prognosis.[36] The 2015 International Atomic Energy Agency (IAEA) consensus report recommended that the interval between staging PET scans and the start of RT should not exceed 3 weeks.[2]

Use of PET for Target Volume Definition in Lung Cancer

When a patient is treated with curative-intent RT, the critical step in treatment planning is the definition of the planning target volume (PTV).[37] The PTV is the volume that will be irradiated to the prescribed tumoricidal radiation dose and it must include all sites of gross tumor with appropriate margins for setup uncertainties and the effects of physiologic movement resulting from respiration and cardiac pulsation. RT target volume definition should ideally be performed using recently acquired FDG/PET-CT images obtained on a modern hybrid scanner, with the patient in the radiotherapy treatment position. Ideally, the setup should be supervised by radiation therapists and all appropriate immobilization devices should be in place. Positioning for PET/CT image acquisition and RT delivery should be identical.[2]

The PTV takes into account the imaged gross tumor volume (GTV); any expansion of the GTV required for movement (producing an internal target volume); and the clinical target volume, which includes suspected microscopic extension beyond the GTV, usually considered to be 5 to 7 mm in NSCLC. The long acquisition time of PET provides information on the average position of the tumor over time. The use of four-dimensional (4D) PET acquisition allows the movement of the tumor to be studied in detail[38–40] and 4D PET can be used to facilitate gated therapy, in which the treatment beam is only turned on when the tumor is in a particular part of the respiratory cycle, thereby reducing the exposure of normal tissues.

The ideal PTV encompasses all tumor sites detected by imaging and biopsy and includes the minimum volume of normal tissues. PET data are critical for contouring both the primary tumor[20] and all involved mediastinal lymph nodes,[41] because of both increased accuracy and greater interobserver reproducibility[42] compared with CT-only contouring. The process of tumor contouring is performed using dedicated RT-planning software with the PET/CT images imported. Window settings for the display of PET/CT images must be carefully defined for each planning system. Images should appear the same on both the PET workstation and the radiotherapy planning workstation. When radiation oncologists draw the edge of the gross tumor, both PET and CT data are considered. The margin of tumor often appears fuzzy on the PET component, making it difficult to consistently define the tumor edge without a systematic approach. The 2016 IAEA report by Konert and colleagues[2] provides detailed guidance on how to define the edge of the tumor for RT planning using a visual approach. Although the use of PET/CT imaging has increased the reproducibility of tumor contouring, because of the superior contrast between tumor and normal tissues compared with CT alone, the best way to derive tumor contours from PET data remains controversial. Visual interpretation and manual contouring of PET-based tumor volumes is the most widely used approach,[43] but a range of different autosegmentation approaches have been developed either to define the tumor volume or to assist with visual contouring.[44] The target volume in modern RT for NSCLC is the generally gross tumor with an appropriate margin.[45] In a pilot trial[46] of PET for target volume delineation, an autocontour was used as the starting point and this is the basis of the current PET-Plan trial. The differing interpretation of mediastinal nodal status could be reduced by a harmonization approach.[47]

The many different autocontouring approaches have been summarized in a recent American Association of Physicists in Medicine (AAPM) report and no single method is suitable in all circumstances.[44] At present, the use of autocontouring is not recommended in routine practice, unless the autocontours are to be used as the basis for subsequent human editing.[48,49] For example, the RTOG 1106 multicenter study defines an FDG-PET metabolic tumor volume using autosegmentation thresholding at 1.5 times the mediastinum blood pool followed by manual editing.[50]

When stereotactic body RT (SBRT) is used to treat small lung tumors, these are typically surrounded by normal lung and are well seen on CT, and 4D CT is used to account for target motion.[51,52] In some cases, three-dimensional (3D) PET information can help with tumor delineation but in most cases the 4D CT is sufficient. The use of 4D PET information in-planning SBRT and conventional RT is an area of active research. For example, the EORTC 2113-0813 Lungtech trial[53,54] is investigating the use of 3D and 4D PET/CT for staging, target delineation, response evaluation, and detecting recurrence in patients treated with SBRT.

There is no randomized evidence supporting the use of PET-based RT planning, largely because the early evidence for the superiority of PET-based staging compared with CT-based staging in lung cancer was so strong. Randomized trials in which some patients would knowingly be randomized to an inferior management strategy are generally considered unethical. The preponderance of evidence from the prospective literature is consistent with a powerful impact of PET on target volume definition, especially with respect to identification of lymph node disease and contouring of primary tumors in cases with atelectasis. There is compelling retrospective evidence that the introduction of CT-based RT planning was associated with a significant improvement in survival in NSCLC compared with two-dimensional imaging.[55] Prospective studies of PET-based planning suggest that outcomes are better still in patients who received curative-intent RT planning with PET data compared with the preceding CT era. Use of PET has been associated with 5-year survival of greater than 30% in stage IIIA NSCLC.[32] These results would have been unheard of in the pre-PET era. However, it is impossible to separately assess the contributions from PET resulting from better staging, patient selection, and RT planning because a single scan can serve all of these purposes.

Response-Adapted Therapy and Targeting of Tumor Subvolumes

The most widely used approach in RT planning for NSCLC is designed to deliver a homogeneous dose to the entire target. However, there is increasing interest in delivery of different RT doses to selected tumor subvolumes, either using baseline PET scan data or interim-response FDG-PET scans performed during the course of RT. The rationale for this is to deliver higher doses to presumably resistant subvolumes either because they contain a greater concentration of presumed resistant tumor cells or because they have been slow to respond. This technique is referred to as dose painting and, in the Netherlands, a PET boost trial it proved feasible to escalate the dose to areas of high initial FDG uptake.[56] Dose painting of hypoxic subvolumes has also been explored.[57] It is not yet clear that survival can be improved using these methods.

Although the original aim of repeated imaging during RT was to ensure that treatment quality was maintained,[58–60] the observation that tumors changed dimensions during RT gave rise to the concept of response-adapted therapy. The rationale for using PET for response assessment in RT-treated patients with NSCLC rather than CT is that FDG uptake in tumors changes more rapidly than tumor volume detected by CT and that response assessment with FDG-PET after completion of RT is superior to CT, both in estimating OS[61] and in predicting patterns of failure.[62] PET-based interim response assessment during RT could potentially provide response information early enough to modify treatment, with dose painting of slowly responding regions, although this is very resource intensive.[63–66]

The best time points for imaging during RT, either for response assessment or for treatment adaptation, are unknown. In one study, early time points, namely 7 days and 14 days into treatment, were used[67] and seemed to offer useful information. Scans performed at around week 4 of RT have been explored by other groups. Later treatment response assessment may be more reliable in predicting outcomes but allows less time for replanning. Interim FDG-PET scans have been used to escalate RT doses in human patients by several groups. For example, Feng and colleagues[68] were able to escalate dose by 30 to 102 Gy (mean, 58 Gy) or reduce the risk of normal tissue complications by 0.4% to 3% in a small cohort when treatment was replanned based on PET/CT response.

A phase II trial was later conducted by this group[69] in which adaptive planning was used after 50 Gy and the RT dosimetry was adapted to target a residual metabolic target volume for 9 fractions. Using an isotoxic approach, the dose per fraction varied between 2.2 and 3.8 Gy for the adaptive part of the treatment.[69] Outcomes seemed to be favorable compared with historical results.

The current RTOG 1106 phase II trial for NSCLC is designed to deliver escalated doses to slow-responding tumors to improve local progression-free survival. FDG-PET response after 18 to 19 treatments is used to help adjust the remaining 9 treatments to boost the residual metabolic tumor volume. Another possible approach could be to select highly PET-responsive tumors for less-intense treatment.

There is potential for using tracers other than FDG for interim response assessment. FDG may accumulate in areas of RT-induced inflammation in normal tissues.[70,71] The most promising alternative approaches include imaging proliferation or hypoxia. Everitt and colleagues[72] studied both FDG and ^{18}F-fluorothymidine (FLT) PET/CT scans during weeks 2 and 4 of chemoRT in 60 patients. An unexpected finding was that stable disease detected on week-2 FLT-PET/CT was associated with longer progression-free survival and OS than with partial or complete reductions in FLT uptake.[30] Progressive proliferative disease was uncommon but was associated with a poor outcome (**Fig. 4**).

Because of bioreductive metabolism in hypoxic tumor regions, hypoxia can be indirectly studied using PET imaging.[73] The tracers ^{18}F-misonadazole (F-MISO) and ^{18}F-fluoroazomycin arabinoside (FAZA)[74] have both been used in humans with lung cancer. Hypoxia, resulting from complex factors, including inadequate tumor vasculature and alterations in tumor cell metabolism, is associated both with local radiation resistance[75] and with increased metastatic potential. Dose painting of radioresistant PET-detected hypoxic subvolumes has the potential to improve results of therapy, especially with 4D acquisition to improve resolution.[74] Vera and colleagues[76] showed differences in the dynamics of F-MISO–PET/CT, FDG-PET/CT, and FLT-PET/CT scans before and after 46 Gy of RT in a small cohort. The hypoxia signal remained stable, whereas the proliferation and metabolism signals declined. Variability of

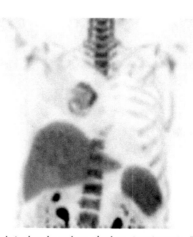

Fig. 4. Interim imaging during treatment. FLT-PET scan of a patient with NSCLC after 4 weeks of a 6-week course of chemoradiation. The scan shows persistent highly proliferative disease and disappearance of the bone marrow signal in regions traversed by the radiation beams. This finding represented an increase in FLT uptake compared with the baseline scan and was associated with early death with local disease progression.

baseline and during-treatment hypoxia burden were observed in a further small study in which F-MISO–PET scans were acquired before, during, and after RT.[77] Trinkaus and colleagues[78] studied FAZA-PET scans in patients with NSCLC and reported that successful RT was associated with disappearance of the hypoxia signal.[78]

IMAGING OF RADIOSENSITIVE NORMAL TISSUES WITH PET

Although the primary role for PET in lung cancer management has been to image the tumor, PET scanning can also give additional information on other biological processes occurring in patients before, during, and after RT, including disorders and toxicities in normal tissues. High-dose thoracic RT is associated with significant toxicity in many cases, especially pneumonitis,[79,80] which has classic radiological and clinical features.

Pneumonitis is associated with increased density[81] and unbalanced enhancement of pulmonary tissue[82] on MR imaging. Radiation pneumonitis is also associated with uptake of FDG in lung and pleura (**Fig. 5**), and FDG-PET imaging may detect abnormalities before symptoms occur.[71] The severity of clinical pneumonitis as assessed by the RTOG grade is significantly correlated with FDG uptake measured by a visual radiotoxicity score on FDG-PET. Detection of FDG uptake in lung during RT has the potential to allow early treatment of pneumonitis or alteration of the RT plan. Sensitive lung perfusion studies with the promising tracer gallium-68 (GalliPET)[83] have shown that early severe reductions in lung perfusion may can be observed within the high-radiation dose volume during treatment.[84] Baseline ventilation and perfusion imaging with GalliPET could potentially be used in RT planning to selectively avoid irradiation of regions of

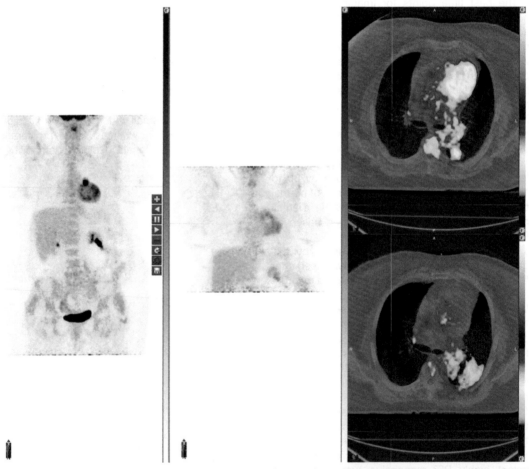

Fig. 5. Pneumonitis detected on FDG-PET. Pretreatment and 2 months posttreatment PET (*left 2 panels*) and PET/CT images from a patient with NSCLC of the left lower lobe treated with curative-intent RT. There has been a complete metabolic response at the primary site but there is intense FDG uptake in previously normal lung, consistent with radiation pneumonitis.

well-perfused[85] and ventilated high-functioning lung and dump excess dose in areas of low-functioning lung that contribute less to respiratory function.

Esophageal toxicity is the most common dose-limiting acute toxicity of chemoRT and can be identified on FDG-PET scans as linear uptake corresponding with the organ.[71,86–91] A linear relationship has been reported between FDG uptake and clinical esophagitis.[87] This information has not yet been shown to have clinical value.

SUMMARY

The planning of curative-intent RT in patients with lung cancer is complex and includes comprehensive assessment of both the tumor and the physiologic status of the patient, including the fitness to undergo therapy. PET imaging, primarily with FDG, plays a critical role in this process. Appropriate patient selection ensures that curative-intent treatment is feasible and that RT, not surgery, is the most appropriate therapy. The presence of comorbidities and the overall performance status of the patient must be considered to ensure that a patient with a likely short survival time is not treated with inappropriately intense therapy. For suitable patients, FDG-PET–based imaging is essential for determining the true stage, supplemented where appropriate by results of EBUS and other investigations. PET/CT is the primary modality for treatment planning in patients with locoregionally advanced disease and has been shown to significantly alter treatment volumes compared with CT-based treatment plans. Patients staged and planned using PET have survival outcomes that are far superior to historical results. Research continues into the use of alternative tracers to FDG, PET-response–adapted therapy, and physiologically guided treatment planning that modifies the dose distribution based on normal tissue imaging. The results of clinical trials that are currently in progress or are in the planning stage will show whether any of these novel approaches will provide further benefits for patients.

ACKNOWLEDGMENTS

Sincere thanks to Dr Tim Akhurst for his assistance with the figures for this article.

REFERENCES

1. Akhurst T, MacManus M, Hicks RJ. Lung cancer. PET Clin 2015;10(2):147–58.
2. Konert T, Vogel W, MacManus MP, et al. PET/CT imaging for target volume delineation in curative intent radiotherapy of non-small cell lung cancer: IAEA consensus report 2014. Radiother Oncol 2015; 116(1):27–34.
3. Murray P, Franks K, Hanna GG. A systematic review of outcomes following stereotactic ablative radiotherapy in the treatment of early-stage primary lung cancer. Br J Radiol 2017;90(1071):20160732.
4. Dingemans AM, de Langen AJ, van den Boogaart V, et al. First-line erlotinib and bevacizumab in patients with locally advanced and/or metastatic non-small-cell lung cancer: a phase II study including molecular imaging. Ann Oncol 2011;22(3):559–66.
5. Eaton BR, Pugh SL, Bradley JD, et al. Institutional enrollment and survival among NSCLC patients receiving chemoradiation: NRG Oncology Radiation Therapy Oncology Group (RTOG) 0617. J Natl Cancer Inst 2016;108(9) [pii:djw034].
6. Chun SG, Hu C, Choy H, et al. Impact of intensity-modulated radiation therapy technique for locally advanced non-small-cell lung cancer: a secondary analysis of the NRG oncology RTOG 0617 randomized clinical trial. J Clin Oncol 2017;35(1):56–62.
7. Goldstraw P, Chansky K, Crowley J, et al. The IASLC Lung Cancer Staging Project: proposals for revision of the TNM stage groupings in the forthcoming (eighth) edition of the TNM classification for lung cancer. J Thorac Oncol 2016;11(1):39–51.
8. Chang JH, Gandhidasan S, Finnigan R, et al. Stereotactic ablative body radiotherapy for the treatment of spinal oligometastases. Clin Oncol 2017;29(7): e119–25.
9. Siva S, Senan S, Ball D. Ablative therapies for lung metastases: a need to acknowledge the efficacy and toxicity of stereotactic ablative body radiotherapy. Ann Oncol 2015;26(10):2196.
10. Alexander M, Evans SM, Stirling RG, et al. The influence of comorbidity and the simplified comorbidity score on overall survival in non-small cell lung cancer–A prospective cohort study. J Thorac Oncol 2016;11(5):748–57.
11. Alexander M, Wolfe R, Ball D, et al. Lung cancer prognostic index: a risk score to predict overall survival after the diagnosis of non-small-cell lung cancer. Br J Cancer 2017;117(5):744–51.
12. Steinfort DP, Siva S, Leong TL, et al. Systematic endobronchial ultrasound-guided mediastinal staging versus positron emission tomography for comprehensive mediastinal staging in NSCLC before radical radiotherapy of non-small cell lung cancer: a pilot study. Medicine 2016;95(8):e2488.
13. Metcalfe P, Liney GP, Holloway L, et al. The potential for an enhanced role for MRI in radiation-therapy treatment planning. Technol Cancer Res Treat 2013;12(5):429–46.
14. Glazer GM, Orringer MB, Gross BH, et al. The mediastinum in non-small cell lung cancer: CT-surgical correlation. AJR Am J Roentgenol 1984;142(6): 1101–5.

15. Andersen MB, Harders SW, Ganeshan B, et al. CT texture analysis can help differentiate between malignant and benign lymph nodes in the mediastinum in patients suspected for lung cancer. Acta Radiol 2016;57(6):669–76.

16. Gould MK, Kuschner WG, Rydzak CE, et al. Test performance of positron emission tomography and computed tomography for mediastinal staging in patients with non-small-cell lung cancer: a meta-analysis. Ann Intern Med 2003;139(11):879–92.

17. Sogaard R, Fischer BM, Mortensen J, et al. Preoperative staging of lung cancer with PET/CT: cost-effectiveness evaluation alongside a randomized controlled trial. Eur J Nucl Med Mol Imaging 2011; 38(5):802–9.

18. Videtic GM, Rice TW, Murthy S, et al. Utility of positron emission tomography compared with mediastinoscopy for delineating involved lymph nodes in stage III lung cancer: insights for radiotherapy planning from a surgical cohort. Int J Radiat Oncol Biol Phys 2008;72(3):702–6.

19. Steinfort DP, Liew D, Irving LB. Radial probe EBUS versus CT-guided needle biopsy for evaluation of peripheral pulmonary lesions: an economic analysis. Eur Respir J 2013;41(3):539–47.

20. Nestle U, Walter K, Schmidt S, et al. 18F-deoxyglucose positron emission tomography (FDG-PET) for the planning of radiotherapy in lung cancer: high impact in patients with atelectasis. Int J Radiat Oncol Biol Phys 1999;44(3):593–7.

21. Mac Manus MP, Hicks RJ, Ball DL, et al. F-18 fluorodeoxyglucose positron emission tomography staging in radical radiotherapy candidates with nonsmall cell lung carcinoma: powerful correlation with survival and high impact on treatment. Cancer 2001;92(4):886–95.

22. Herder GJ, Golding RP, Hoekstra OS, et al. The performance of (18)F-fluorodeoxyglucose positron emission tomography in small solitary pulmonary nodules. Eur J Nucl Med Mol Imaging 2004;31(9): 1231–6.

23. Louie AV, Senan S, Patel P, et al. When is a biopsy-proven diagnosis necessary before stereotactic ablative radiotherapy for lung cancer?: a decision analysis. Chest 2014;146(4):1021–8.

24. Seute T, Leffers P, ten Velde GP, et al. Detection of brain metastases from small cell lung cancer: consequences of changing imaging techniques (CT versus MRI). Cancer 2008;112(8):1827–34.

25. Hjorthaug K, Hojbjerg JA, Knap MM, et al. Accuracy of 18F-FDG PET-CT in triaging lung cancer patients with suspected brain metastases for MRI. Nucl Med Commun 2015;36(11):1084–90.

26. MacManus MP, Hicks RJ, Matthews JP, et al. High rate of detection of unsuspected distant metastases by pet in apparent stage III non-small-cell lung cancer: implications for radical radiation therapy. Int J Radiat Oncol Biol Phys 2001;50(2): 287–93.

27. Yun M, Kim W, Alnafisi N, et al. 18F-FDG PET in characterizing adrenal lesions detected on CT or MRI. J Nucl Med 2001;42(12):1795–9.

28. Bury T, Barreto A, Daenen F, et al. Fluorine-18 deoxyglucose positron emission tomography for the detection of bone metastases in patients with non-small cell lung cancer. Eur J Nucl Med 1998;25(9): 1244–7.

29. Grassetto G, Fornasiero A, Bonciarelli G, et al. Additional value of FDG-PET/CT in management of "solitary" liver metastases: preliminary results of a prospective multicenter study. Mol Imaging Biol 2010;12(2):139–44.

30. Ball D, Everitt S, Hicks R, et al. Serial FDG and FLT PET/CT during curative-intent chemo-radiotherapy for NSCLC impacts patient management and may predict clinical outcomes. J Thorac Oncol 2017; 12(1):S420.

31. Mac Manus MP, Wong K, Hicks RJ, et al. Early mortality after radical radiotherapy for non-small-cell lung cancer: comparison of PET-staged and conventionally staged cohorts treated at a large tertiary referral center. Int J Radiat Oncol Biol Phys 2002;52(2):351–61.

32. Mac Manus MP, Everitt S, Bayne M, et al. The use of fused PET/CT images for patient selection and radical radiotherapy target volume definition in patients with non-small cell lung cancer: results of a prospective study with mature survival data. Radiother Oncol 2013;106(3):292–8.

33. Kolodziejczyk M, Kepka L, Dziuk M, et al. Impact of [18F]fluorodeoxyglucose PET-CT staging on treatment planning in radiotherapy incorporating elective nodal irradiation for non-small-cell lung cancer: a prospective study. Int J Radiat Oncol Biol Phys 2011;80(4):1008–14.

34. Geiger GA, Kim MB, Xanthopoulos EP, et al. Stage migration in planning PET/CT scans in patients due to receive radiotherapy for non-small-cell lung cancer. Clin Lung Cancer 2014;15(1):79–85.

35. Everitt S, Herschtal A, Callahan J, et al. High rates of tumor growth and disease progression detected on serial pretreatment fluorodeoxyglucose-positron emission tomography/computed tomography scans in radical radiotherapy candidates with nonsmall cell lung cancer. Cancer 2010;116(21):5030–7.

36. Everitt S, Plumridge N, Herschtal A, et al. The impact of time between staging PET/CT and definitive chemo-radiation on target volumes and survival in patients with non-small cell lung cancer. Radiother Oncol 2013;106(3):288–91.

37. Gregoire V, Mackie TR. State of the art on dose prescription, reporting and recording in intensity-modulated radiation therapy (ICRU report no. 83). Cancer Radiother 2011;15(6–7):555–9.

38. Chirindel A, Adebahr S, Schuster D, et al. Impact of 4D-(18)FDG-PET/CT imaging on target volume delineation in SBRT patients with central versus peripheral lung tumors. Multi-reader comparative study. Radiother Oncol 2015;115(3):335–41.

39. Callahan J, Kron T, Siva S, et al. Geographic miss of lung tumours due to respiratory motion: a comparison of 3D vs 4D PET/CT defined target volumes. Radiat Oncol 2014;9:291.

40. Sindoni A, Minutoli F, Pontoriero A, et al. Usefulness of four dimensional (4D) PET/CT imaging in the evaluation of thoracic lesions and in radiotherapy planning: review of the literature. Lung cancer 2016;96:78–86.

41. De Ruysscher D, Wanders S, van Haren E, et al. Selective mediastinal node irradiation based on FDG-PET scan data in patients with non-small-cell lung cancer: a prospective clinical study. Int J Radiat Oncol Biol Phys 2005;62(4):988–94.

42. Caldwell CB, Mah K, Ung YC, et al. Observer variation in contouring gross tumor volume in patients with poorly defined non-small-cell lung tumors on CT: the impact of 18FDG-hybrid PET fusion. Int J Radiat Oncol Biol Phys 2001;51(4):923–31.

43. Werner-Wasik M, Nelson AD, Choi W, et al. What is the best way to contour lung tumors on PET scans? Multiobserver validation of a gradient-based method using a NSCLC digital PET phantom. Int J Radiat Oncol Biol Phys 2012;82(3):1164–71.

44. Hatt M, Lee JA, Schmidtlein CR, et al. Classification and evaluation strategies of auto-segmentation approaches for PET: report of AAPM task group No. 211. Med Phys 2017;44(6):e1–42.

45. De Ruysscher D, Wanders S, Minken A, et al. Effects of radiotherapy planning with a dedicated combined PET-CT-simulator of patients with non-small cell lung cancer on dose limiting normal tissues and radiation dose-escalation: a planning study. Radiother Oncol 2005;77(1):5–10.

46. Fleckenstein J, Hellwig D, Kremp S, et al. F-18-FDG-PET confined radiotherapy of locally advanced NSCLC with concomitant chemotherapy: results of the PET-PLAN pilot trial. Int J Radiat Oncol Biol Phys 2011;81(4):e283–9.

47. Nestle U, Rischke HC, Eschmann SM, et al. Improved inter-observer agreement of an expert review panel in an oncology treatment trial–Insights from a structured interventional process. Eur J Cancer 2015;51(17):2525–33.

48. MacManus M, Nestle U, Rosenzweig KE, et al. Use of PET and PET/CT for radiation therapy planning: IAEA expert report 2006-2007. Radiother Oncol 2009;91(1):85–94.

49. Doll C, Duncker-Rohr V, Rucker G, et al. Influence of experience and qualification on PET-based target volume delineation. When there is no expert–ask your colleague. Strahlenther Onkol 2014;190(6):555–62.

50. Mahasittiwat P, Yuan S, Xie C, et al. Metabolic tumor volume on PET reduced more than gross tumor volume on CT during radiotherapy in patients with non-small cell lung cancer treated with 3DCRT or SBRT. J Radiat Oncol 2013;2(2):191–202.

51. Brandner ED, Chetty IJ, Giaddui TG, et al. Motion management strategies and technical issues associated with stereotactic body radiotherapy of thoracic and upper abdominal tumors: a review from NRG oncology. Med Phys 2017;44(6):2595–612.

52. De Ruysscher D, Faivre-Finn C, Nestle U, et al. European Organisation for Research and Treatment of Cancer recommendations for planning and delivery of high-dose, high-precision radiotherapy for lung cancer. J Clin Oncol 2010;28(36):5301–10.

53. Adebahr S, Collette S, Shash E, et al. LungTech, an EORTC phase II trial of stereotactic body radiotherapy for centrally located lung tumours: a clinical perspective. Br J Radiol 2015;88(1051):20150036.

54. Lambrecht M, Melidis C, Sonke JJ, et al. Lungtech, a phase II EORTC trial of SBRT for centrally located lung tumours - a clinical physics perspective. Radiat Oncol 2016;11:7.

55. Chen AB, Neville BA, Sher DJ, et al. Survival outcomes after radiation therapy for stage III non-small-cell lung cancer after adoption of computed tomography-based simulation. J Clin Oncol 2011;29(17):2305–11.

56. van Elmpt W, De Ruysscher D, van der Salm A, et al. The PET-boost randomised phase II dose-escalation trial in non-small cell lung cancer. Radiother Oncol 2012;104(1):67–71.

57. Even AJ, van der Stoep J, Zegers CM, et al. PET-based dose painting in non-small cell lung cancer: comparing uniform dose escalation with boosting hypoxic and metabolically active sub-volumes. Radiother Oncol 2015;116(2):281–6.

58. Yan D, Lockman D, Martinez A, et al. Computed tomography guided management of interfractional patient variation. Semin Radiat Oncol 2005;15(3):168–79.

59. Li XA, Qi XS, Pitterle M, et al. Interfractional variations in patient setup and anatomic change assessed by daily computed tomography. Int J Radiat Oncol Biol Phys 2007;68(2):581–91.

60. Hugo GD, Yan D, Liang J. Population and patient-specific target margins for 4D adaptive radiotherapy to account for intra- and inter-fraction variation in lung tumour position. Phys Med Biol 2007;52(1):257–74.

61. Mac Manus MP, Hicks RJ, Matthews JP, et al. Positron emission tomography is superior to computed tomography scanning for response-assessment after radical radiotherapy or chemoradiotherapy in

patients with non-small-cell lung cancer. J Clin Oncol 2003;21(7):1285–92.

62. Mac Manus MP, Hicks RJ, Matthews JP, et al. Metabolic (FDG-PET) response after radical radiotherapy/chemoradiotherapy for non-small cell lung cancer correlates with patterns of failure. Lung cancer 2005;49(1):95–108.

63. Jaffray DA, Siewerdsen JH, Wong JW, et al. Flat-panel cone-beam computed tomography for image-guided radiation therapy. Int J Radiat Oncol Biol Phys 2002;53(5):1337–49.

64. Nielsen M, Bertelsen A, Westberg J, et al. Cone beam CT evaluation of patient set-up accuracy as a QA tool. Acta Oncol 2009;48(2):271–6.

65. Jaffray DA, Drake DG, Moreau M, et al. A radiographic and tomographic imaging system integrated into a medical linear accelerator for localization of bone and soft-tissue targets. Int J Radiat Oncol Biol Phys 1999;45(3):773–89.

66. Sorcini B, Tilikidis A. Clinical application of image-guided radiotherapy, IGRT (on the Varian OBI platform). Cancer Radiother 2006;10(5):252–7.

67. van Baardwijk A, Bosmans G, Dekker A, et al. Time trends in the maximal uptake of FDG on PET scan during thoracic radiotherapy. A prospective study in locally advanced non-small cell lung cancer (NSCLC) patients. Radiother Oncol 2007;82(2):145–52.

68. Feng M, Kong FM, Gross M, et al. Using fluorodeoxyglucose positron emission tomography to assess tumor volume during radiotherapy for non-small-cell lung cancer and its potential impact on adaptive dose escalation and normal tissue sparing. Int J Radiat Oncol Biol Phys 2009;73(4):1228–34.

69. Kong FM, Ten Haken RK, Schipper MJ, et al. A phase II trial of mid-treatment FDG-PET adaptive, individualized radiation therapy plus concurrent chemotherapy in patients with non-small cell lung cancer (NSCLC). 2013 ASCO Annual Meeting. J Clin Oncol 2013;31(Suppl) [abstract: 7522].

70. Bollineni VR, Widder J, Pruim J, et al. Residual 18F-FDG-PET uptake 12 weeks after stereotactic ablative radiotherapy for stage I non-small-cell lung cancer predicts local control. Int J Radiat Oncol Biol Phys 2012;83(4):e551–5.

71. Mac Manus MP, Ding Z, Hogg A, et al. Association between pulmonary uptake of fluorodeoxyglucose detected by positron emission tomography scanning after radiation therapy for non-small-cell lung cancer and radiation pneumonitis. Int J Radiat Oncol Biol Phys 2011;80(5):1365–71.

72. Everitt SJ, Ball DL, Hicks RJ, et al. Differential (18)F-FDG and (18)F-FLT uptake on serial PET/CT imaging before and during definitive chemoradiation for non-small cell lung cancer. J Nucl Med 2014;55(7):1069–74.

73. Bollineni VR, Wiegman EM, Pruim J, et al. Hypoxia imaging using positron emission tomography in non-small cell lung cancer: implications for radiotherapy. Cancer Treat Rev 2012;38(8):1027–32.

74. Bollineni VR, Kerner GS, Pruim J, et al. PET imaging of tumor hypoxia using 18F-fluoroazomycin arabinoside in stage III-IV non-small cell lung cancer patients. J Nucl Med 2013;54(8):1175–80.

75. Deschner EE, Gray LH. Influence of oxygen tension on x-ray-induced chromosomal damage in Ehrlich ascites tumor cells irradiated in vitro and in vivo. Radiat Res 1959;11(1):115–46.

76. Vera P, Bohn P, Edet-Sanson A, et al. Simultaneous positron emission tomography (PET) assessment of metabolism with 18F-fluoro-2-deoxy-d-glucose (FDG), proliferation with 18F-fluoro-thymidine (FLT), and hypoxia with 18fluoro-misonidazole (F-miso) before and during radiotherapy in patients with non-small-cell lung cancer (NSCLC): a pilot study. Radiother Oncol 2011;98(1):109–16.

77. Koh WJ, Bergman KS, Rasey JS, et al. Evaluation of oxygenation status during fractionated radiotherapy in human nonsmall cell lung cancers using [F-18]fluoromisonidazole positron emission tomography. Int J Radiat Oncol Biol Phys 1995;33(2):391–8.

78. Trinkaus ME, Blum R, Rischin D, et al. Imaging of hypoxia with 18F-FAZA PET in patients with locally advanced non-small cell lung cancer treated with definitive chemoradiotherapy. J Med Imaging Radiat Oncol 2013;57(4):475–81.

79. Mah K, Van Dyk J, Keane T, et al. Acute radiation-induced pulmonary damage: a clinical study on the response to fractionated radiation therapy. Int J Radiat Oncol Biol Phys 1987;13(2):179–88.

80. Boersma LJ, Damen EM, de Boer RW, et al. Recovery of overall and local lung function loss 18 months after irradiation for malignant lymphoma. J Clin Oncol 1996;14(5):1431–41.

81. Yankelevitz DF, Henschke CI, Batata M, et al. Lung cancer: evaluation with MR imaging during and after irradiation. J Thorac Imaging 1994;9(1):41–6.

82. Ogasawara N, Suga K, Karino Y, et al. Perfusion characteristics of radiation-injured lung on Gd-DTPA-enhanced dynamic magnetic resonance imaging. Invest Radiol 2002;37(8):448–57.

83. Siva S, Callahan J, Kron T, et al. A prospective observational study of gallium-68 ventilation and perfusion PET/CT during and after radiotherapy in patients with non-small cell lung cancer. BMC Cancer 2014;14:740.

84. Siva S, Hardcastle N, Kron T, et al. Ventilation/perfusion positron emission tomography–based assessment of radiation injury to lung. Int J Radiat Oncol Biol Phys 2015;93(2):408–17.

85. Siva S, Thomas R, Callahan J, et al. High-resolution pulmonary ventilation and perfusion PET/CT allows

for functionally adapted intensity modulated radiotherapy in lung cancer. Radiother Oncol 2015; 115(2):157–62.

86. Hicks RJ, Mac Manus MP, Matthews JP, et al. Early FDG-PET imaging after radical radiotherapy for non-small-cell lung cancer: inflammatory changes in normal tissues correlate with tumor response and do not confound therapeutic response evaluation. Int J Radiat Oncol Biol Phys 2004;60(2):412–8.

87. Guerrero T, Johnson V, Hart J, et al. Radiation pneumonitis: local dose versus [18F]-fluorodeoxyglucose uptake response in irradiated lung. Int J Radiat Oncol Biol Phys 2007;68(4):1030–5.

88. Hart JP, McCurdy MR, Ezhil M, et al. Radiation pneumonitis: correlation of toxicity with pulmonary metabolic radiation response. Int J Radiat Oncol Biol Phys 2008;71(4):967–71.

89. Abdulla S, Salavati A, Saboury B, et al. Quantitative assessment of global lung inflammation following radiation therapy using FDG PET/CT: a pilot study. Eur J Nucl Med Mol Imaging 2014; 41(2):350–6.

90. McCurdy M, Bergsma DP, Hyun E, et al. The role of lung lobes in radiation pneumonitis and radiation-induced inflammation in the lung: a retrospective study. J Radiat Oncol 2013;2(2): 203–8.

91. McCurdy MR, Castillo R, Martinez J, et al. [18F]-FDG uptake dose-response correlates with radiation pneumonitis in lung cancer patients. Radiother Oncol 2012;104(1):52–7.

Prognostic Value of ^{18}F-Fluorodeoxyglucose PET/Computed Tomography in Non–Small-Cell Lung Cancer

CrossMark

Gang Cheng, MD, PhD[a],*, He Huang, MD[b]

KEYWORDS

- Non–small-cell lung cancer • FDG-PET/CT • FDG uptake • Prognosis • Survival

KEY POINTS

- The tumor-node-metastasis (TNM) staging system is the most important prognostic indicator in primary non–small-cell lung cancer (NSCLC). Other important prognostic factors include performance status, weight loss, proliferation level, and other tumor biology features.
- ^{18}F-Fluorodeoxyglucose uptake, reflecting tissue metabolic activity, is an important aspect of tumor biology. Multiple studies have shown the predictive and prognostic values of maximum standardized uptake value (SUV_{max}) from the primary tumor in patients with NSCLC at initial diagnosis, after induction therapy, and in posttreatment patients.
- The prognostic value of SUV_{max} in NSCLC seems to be independent of treatment received, tumor staging, tumor histology, and other factors.
- Volume-based PET parameters such as metabolic tumor volume and total lesion glycolysis, which represent FDG activity in the entire tumor mass, reflect the metabolic status of a malignancy more accurately than SUV_{max}, and thus are better prognostic markers in lung cancer.
- Volume-based PET parameters were shown to be significant prognosticators in NSCLC survival even when SUV_{max} was not.
- The incorporation of quantitative FDG activity in tumor staging and therapy response criteria in the future may allow better risk stratification and better treatment outcomes.

Lung cancer remains a leading cause of cancer-related deaths worldwide, accounting for approximately 224,390 new patients and 158,080 deaths in 2016, according to the American Cancer Society.[1] Non–small-cell lung cancer (NSCLC) accounts for approximately 85% of all lung cancers. Approximately 15% to 20% of patients with NSCLC with early-stage, localized disease are amenable to curative surgical resection, which bears the best prognosis; however, multidisciplinary therapy, such as chemoradiotherapy, is becoming increasingly important in patients with more advanced NSCLC who have unresectable tumors or cannot tolerate surgery.[2] Despite significant advances in both diagnostic and therapeutic approaches, the prognosis of patients with lung cancer with regional or distant metastases remain poor.[3] Small cell lung cancer (SCLC) accounts for 13% to 20% of all lung cancers and is a fast-growing aggressive malignancy

Disclosure: None.
[a] Department of Radiology, Hospital of the University of Pennsylvania, 3400 Spruce Street, Philadelphia, PA 19104, USA; [b] Department of Nuclear Medicine, Luzhou People's Hospital, Luzhou, Sichuan Province, People's Republic of China
* Corresponding author.
E-mail address: gang.cheng@uphs.upenn.edu

PET Clin 13 (2018) 59–72
https://doi.org/10.1016/j.cpet.2017.08.006
1556-8598/18/Published by Elsevier Inc.

pet.theclinics.com

with a rapid doubling time, high prevalence of metastatic disease, and very poor prognosis.

Accurate cancer staging is critical for optimal treatment. Traditionally, computed tomography (CT) has been the major imaging modality for NSCLC staging. Over the last 10 years, ^{18}F-fluorodeoxyglucose (FDG) PET/CT has established its value in cancer imaging for a variety of malignancies, including lung cancer.[4] FDG-PET/CT allows the detection of unexpected malignant lesions during initial staging and early detection of recurrence and metastatic spread during restaging. As a marker of glycolysis, the metabolic information provided by FDG-PET can be used to distinguish fibrosis and scarring from residual viable tumors after therapy, independent of anatomic changes in tumor mass. PET/CT has become the standard imaging modality for lung nodule characterization,[5] as well as for lung cancer initial staging,[6,7] treatment planning, treatment response assessment,[8] restaging at recurrence,[9,10] and surveillance.[11] The wide clinical adoption of FDG-PET/CT in patients with lung cancer has improved staging and restaging accuracy, allowing better treatment planning and better evaluation of response to treatment.

One of the major challenges in the management of patients with lung cancer is poor treatment outcome. It is well known that lung cancer is associated with poor prognosis, especially for advanced stages, having only slightly improved despite the development of therapeutic methods and agents in the last few decades. Understanding the prognosis of lung cancer is critically important for patient management. Although undertreatment may be an important cause of treatment failure or tumor recurrence, overtreatment may cause severe side effects and body damage.

The tumor-node-metastasis (TNM) staging system is the most important prognostic indicator in guiding treatment decisions in primary NSCLC.[12] However, the TNM staging system is mainly based on anatomic findings, lacks a biological profile of NSCLC, and as a result does not provide a satisfactory explanation for differences in recurrence and survival in apparently similarly staged patients. Specifically, the TNM staging system does not provide tumor-specific and patient-specific characteristics in patients with the same disease stage. It is often noted that patients with NSCLC within the same stage with similar pathologic features show variable responses and survival rates, even with similar treatment. In addition to tumor stage at presentation, many other factors have been used to predict the biological behavior of NSCLC, including performance status,[13–17] weight loss,[18–20] proliferation,[21] histology,[22] and

various molecular markers.[23] This article discusses the value of FDG activity as a prognostic indicator in patients with NSCLC.

MAXIMUM STANDARDIZED UPTAKE VALUE AS A NON–SMALL-CELL LUNG CANCER PROGNOSTICATOR

The standardized uptake value (SUV) is commonly used as a semiquantitative measurement of FDG uptake, representing the radioactivity concentration as measured by the PET scanner within a region of interest (ROI) divided by patient body weight. Maximum SUV (SUV_{max}) quantifies FDG uptake in the voxel containing the maximum FDG activity within an ROI. SUV_{max} is the most commonly used method in clinical practice and is generally accepted as a semiquantitative indicator of a neoplasm's glucose metabolism, because it is easy to calculate. Numerous studies have shown the predictive and prognostic value of SUV_{max} from the primary tumor in patients with NSCLC at initial diagnosis,[14,22,24–27] after induction therapy,[28–30] and in posttreatment.[31,32]

Pretreatment Maximum Standardized Uptake Value

Preoperative maximum standardized uptake value

Murakami and colleagues[33] evaluated the prognostic value of preoperative FDG-PET in 100 patients with pathologic stage IA lung adenocarcinoma who underwent complete resection. Preoperative SUV_{max} was significantly correlated with recurrence and time to recurrence. Three-year disease-free survival (DFS) rates were 97.1% in solid-type adenocarcinomas with SUV_{max} less than 2.15, and 74.1% in solid-type adenocarcinoma with SUV_{max} greater than or equal to 2.15. Similar findings were reported by other researchers.[34–36]

Memorial Sloan Kettering Cancer Center reported a retrospective review involving more advanced NSCLC (T1–T4, N0–N2, M0), indicating that, in surgically managed patients with lung cancer, SUV_{max} was a predictor of overall survival (OS) after resection. The study included 100 consecutive patients (48 men and 52 women) with histologically proven NSCLC or carcinoid pathologic treated by R0 resection (87 patients had lobectomy, others received wedge or segmentectomy, bilobectomy, and pneumonectomy), with no neoadjuvant or adjuvant therapy. These patients had no metachronous lung cancers treated for at least 2 years before or after the study period, and had a follow-up for survival analysis of at least 16 months (median follow-up, 28 months; range, 16–81 months). SUV_{max} analyzed as a continuous variable was significantly correlated with survival. The 2-year survival was 68% for patients with SUV_{max} more than 9 and 96% for those with SUV_{max} less than 9 ($P<.01$). Patients with both T less than 3 cm and SUV_{max} less than 9 had a 3-year survival of 97%, in contrast with 47% in patients with T more than 3 cm and SUV_{max} more than 9 ($P<.01$).[22]

Preradiation maximum standardized uptake value

Multiple studies show that pretreatment SUV_{max} predicts therapeutic outcome in patients with NSCLC treated with stereotactic body radiation therapy (SBRT).[16,37–39] Horne and colleagues[16] evaluated correlation between pretreatment SUV_{max} and progression-free survival (PFS) in early-stage (T1a–T2a, according to the American Joint Committee on Cancer, Seventh Edition) primary NSCLC treated with SBRT in a total of 95 patients with biopsy-confirmed NSCLC. With a median follow-up time of 16 months (range, 1–63 months), these patients had a median OS and PFS of 25.3 months and 40.3 months, respectively. For dichotomous univariate analyses using an SUV of 5 as a cutoff, SUV_{max} predicted for OS and PFS ($P = .024$ for each), although it did not achieve significance for local control (LC) ($P = .256$), regional control (RC) ($P = .131$), or distant control (DC) ($P = .371$). If analyzed as a continuous variable, SUV_{max} predicted for OS ($P = .032$; HR $= 1.061$), PFS ($P = .003$; HR $= 1.098$), and LC ($P = .045$; HR $= 1.124$).[16]

Clarke and colleagues[39] reported that pretreatment SUV_{max} on FDG-PET/CT predicted SBRT outcomes in 82 consecutive patients with medically inoperable early-stage NSCLC, with median follow-up of 2 years. On univariate analysis, pretreatment SUV_{max} predicted for distant failure ($P = .0096$), local failure ($P = .044$), and relapse-free survival (RFS) ($P = .037$). On multivariate analysis pretreatment SUV_{max} predicted for RFS ($P = .037$). Pretreatment SUV_{max} of more than 5 was the most statistically significant cutoff point for predicting distant failure ($P = .0002$). The investigators also reported that patients with a post-SBRT SUV_{max} greater than 2 and a reduction of less than 2.55 had a significantly higher rate of distant failure.[39]

Prechemotherapy maximum standardized uptake value

Imamura and colleagues[40] showed that, using cutoff value of 6.0, pretreatment SUV_{max} had a significant impact on PFS ($P = .008$) and OS ($P = .045$) in patients with NSCLC who received chemotherapy, which was independent of other clinical factors, such as histology and stage.

Posttreatment Maximum Standardized Uptake Value as an Non–Small-Cell Lung Cancer Prognosticator

Treatment of NSCLC by surgery alone often leads to disappointing survival outcomes, because preoperative clinical stage often differs from pathologic findings. Induction chemotherapy before surgery is often used in patients with N2 lymph node metastases or with large T lesions, to produce tumor downstaging that increases the likelihood of complete resection and long-term survival. In addition to SUV in pretreatment primary lung cancer, SUV_{max} in intratreatment FDG-PET/CT shows prognostic value for early treatment response prediction and patient survival. Multiple studies suggest that changes in FDG activity in the primary site of lung cancer during induction therapy or during interim measurement, measured by changes in SUV from baseline, correlate with tumor response and treatment outcome,[41–47] although discrepancies exist.[48]

Maximum standardized uptake value in postinduction/early response

Various studies have also reported that the change in SUV before and after variable chemotherapy is significantly associated with the outcome in patients with NSCLC, allowing for treatment adjustment according to the tumor response in individual patients.[42,44,46,49] Kim and colleagues[44] evaluated the prognostic value of FDG activity after induction chemotherapy in patients with locally advanced NSCLC. The study included 42 cases of clinical stage IIIA-N2 NSCLC, all having received 2 to 4 cycles of preoperative chemotherapy with or without radiation followed by curative surgery. Complete responders on FDG-PET after induction chemotherapy had a significantly longer RFS time than did incomplete responders (28.3 vs 9.1 months; $P = .021$), indicating FDG activity as a good prognosticator for RFS in patients with stage IIIA-N2 NSCLC who received surgery with or without radiation.

Most studies of prognostic value of pretreatment FDG activity were focused on primary lung lesion. However, mediastinal node uptake in post-treatment patients may also bear prognostic significance. Kamel and colleagues[47] analyzed 203 patients with stage IIIA N2 NSCLC who underwent potentially curative lung resection after induction therapy. The median time from completion of chemotherapy to repeat postinduction PET scan was 0.77 months, and the median time from completion of induction therapy to surgical resection was 1.21 months. The postsurgical pathology confirmed that 52% had persistent N2 disease. Factors associated with persistent mediastinal nodal metastasis on univariate analysis included the number of PET-positive N2 stations after induction therapy, the SUV_{max} of N2 nodes on post-induction PET, and whether there was less than a 60% reduction in SUV_{max} of mediastinal lymph nodes. On multivariable analysis, the less than 60% reduction in mediastinal nodal SUV_{max} after induction therapy was found to be an independent predictor of persistent mediastinal nodal metastasis ($P = .037$), which is often associated with poor survival rates.

Maximum standardized uptake value postradiation/posttreatment

MD Anderson Cancer Center studied the efficacy of SUV_{max} in predicting clinical outcome for patients with stage III NSCLC treated prospectively with proton therapy and concurrent chemotherapy. The study included 84 patients with a median follow-up time of 19.2 months (range, 6.1–52.4 months). SUV_{max} values of the primary tumor were obtained from pretreatment ($SUV_{max}1$) and posttreatment ($SUV_{max}2$) PET/CT scans, taken within 6 months of each other. Multivariate analysis showed that Karnofsky performance status (KPS) and $SUV_{max}2$ (cutoff value of 3.6, the median) were independently prognostic for local recurrence-free survival (LRFS), whereas $SUV_{max}1$ (cutoff value of ≥14.2, the median), $SUV_{max}2$, and KPS were independently prognostic for distant metastasis-free survival (DMFS), PFS, and OS ($P<.05$) in patients with stage III NSCLC treated with concurrent chemotherapy and high-dose proton therapy.[50] In a multicenter, prospective National Cancer Institute–funded American College of Radiology Imaging Network (ACRIN)/Radiation Therapy Oncology Group cooperative group trial, the investigators evaluated the correlation between SUVs on posttreatment FDG-PET with survival in patients with stage III NSCLC who received conventional concurrent platinum-based chemo-radiotherapy without surgery. The study involved 226 patients evaluable for pretreatment SUV analysis and 173 patients evaluable for posttreatment SUV analyses (posttreatment FDG-PET was performed at approximately 14 weeks after radiotherapy). Higher posttreatment tumor SUV (peak SUV [SUV_{peak}] or SUV_{max}) was associated with worse survival in stage III NSCLC.[51]

Maximum Standardized Uptake Value Controversies

Many investigators have reported on the function of SUV_{max} in primary lung malignancy as a prognosis indicator.[37–39,52] However, other studies failed to find a correlation between pretreatment SUV_{max} and subsequent tumor response to treatment or survival in patients with NSCLC.[52–56]

Ikushima and colleagues[52] evaluated the relationship between SUV_{max} and clinical tumor features (local-regional recurrence, distant metastases, and survival) in 149 patients with NSCLC. These patients underwent pretreatment PET or PET/CT and were treated with definitive radiotherapy. SUV_{max} was not a consistently significant predictor of tumor recurrence and survival after radiotherapy: a low SUV_{max} was a significant positive factor for locoregional control (LRC), DMFS, and OS on univariate analysis in the PET-alone group, but this significance decreased in multivariate analysis with the inclusion of tumor size. Furthermore, a high SUV_{max} was not a negative factor for LRC, DMFS, or OS on either univariate analysis or multivariate analysis in the PET/CT group.

Vesselle and colleagues[57] prospectively evaluated the prognostic significance of FDG uptake in 208 potentially patients with resectable NSCLC, followed for a median of 33.6 months. SUV_{max} (cutoff value of 7) was significantly associated with an increased risk of death from NSCLC in univariable analysis, whereas the SUV_{max} partial volume corrected for lesion size ($PVCSUV_{max}$) was only marginally associated with survival. In addition, in multivariable analyses, neither SUV_{max} nor $PVCSUV_{max}$ provided significant additional prognostic information over stage, tumor size, and age.

The failure of SUV_{max} as a prognostic factor for NSCLC survival to reach statistically significant levels in these studies may have a variety of underlying causes. It was suspected that small sample size, SUV assessment method, heterogeneity in tumor staging and histology, and treatment strategy may contribute to such findings.[16]

Despite these contradictory results, most studies supported the prognostic value of SUV in patients with lung cancer, as shown by positive findings in recent meta-analyses. The International Association for the Study of Lung Cancer (IASLC) conducted a meta-analysis (including 21 studies, 2637 patients) and found that primary tumor SUV_{max} before any treatment is a significant prognosticator for OS in patients with NSCLC. Patients with a tumor with a higher SUV have shorter survival than patients with a tumor with a lower SUV. Using the median SUV value of each study as threshold, the investigators found a significant prognostic value for high SUV compared with low SUV with an overall combined hazard ratio (HR) of 2.08 (95% confidence interval [CI], 1.69–2.56).[58] Similar findings have been reported in more recent meta-analyses in either patients with surgically treated NSCLC[59] or in patients treated with SBRT.[60]

VOLUME-BASED PET PARAMETERS: BETTER PROGNOSTICATORS

One important concern with SUV_{max} is its quantification of FDG activity from a single hot pixel within a tumor mass, which does not necessarily represent the metabolic status of the tumor. This concern is especially important if the tumor has a highly heterogeneous FDG activity and if most of the tumor mass has SUV much lower than the SUV_{max} obtained. In addition, SUV_{max} can vary secondarily to uptake time, patient obesity, blood glucose level, image noise, methods of attenuation correction, and reconstruction.

To overcome the limitations of SUV_{max}, volume-based PET parameters such as metabolic tumor volume (MTV) and total lesion glycolysis (TLG) have been used. MTV measures tumor volume in voxels to correspond with the volume of metabolically active tumor mass, and is estimated by a semiautomatic tumor-contouring software with a predefined SUV as a threshold (often 40%–50% of SUV_{max}) to segment metabolic tumor boundaries. TLG is the product of the MTV and associated mean SUV (SUV_{mean}). Although SUV_{max} represents the FDG activity of a single pixel, volume-based PET parameters evaluate FDG activity in the entire tumor mass. MTV and TLG may be used to estimate FDG activity in the entire body to determine the total tumor burden in a patient, because the MTV and TLG from multiple lesions can be summed. As a result, MTV and TLG are thought to more accurately reflect the metabolic status of a malignancy than SUV_{max}, and thus are considered better prognostic markers in a variety of types of malignancies, including lung cancer.

Pretreatment Metabolic Tumor Volume and Total Lesion Glycolysis are Prognostic

Analysis of the prospective ACRIN 6668/Radiation Therapy Oncology Group 0235 trial showed that higher pretreatment MTV (tMTV-pre) was associated with significantly worse OS in inoperable stage III NSCLC treated with definitive chemoradiation therapy (CRT). The study included 230 patients with medically inoperable stage III (or selected inoperable stage IIB) NSCLC who received pretreatment FDG-PET scans and were treated with definitive CRT. Patients with higher pretreatment MTV (>32 mL; median value) had worse median OS (14.8 vs 29.7 months; $P<.001$) than patients with lower pretreatment MTV (<32 mL). Every 10-mL increase in tMTV-pre was associated with a 3% increase in risk of death ($P<.001$), after controlling for other variables. On multivariate analysis, tMTV-pre was significantly associated with OS ($P<.001$).[61]

Chung and colleagues[62] investigated MTV and TLG as prognostic factors in 106 patients with newly diagnosed, biopsy-confirmed lung adenocarcinoma (19 stage I/II and 87 stage III/IV lung adenocarcinoma) who underwent FDG-PET/CT before treatment. These patients had no previously known history of cancer. Of these patients, 39.6% (42 out of 106) had epidermal growth factor receptor (EGFR) mutations. Patients with brain metastasis were excluded from the study because torso FDG-PET/CT images were used for the analysis of volume-based parameters. Whole MTV and whole TLG represented the summation of the MTV and TLG values of all lesions in each patient. These patients received surgery, chemotherapy, and/or radiotherapy according to the type and stage of tumor and their medical conditions. Advanced stage (≥III) and poor Eastern Cooperative Oncology Group (ECOG) performance status (≥2) were significant predictors of poor PFS and poor OS. In addition, univariate survival analysis found that high whole MTV (≥90) and high whole TLG (≥600) were significant predictors of poor PFS, whereas high whole MTV (≥90), high whole TLG (≥600), and EGFR mutation–negative status were significant predictors of poor OS. Multivariate survival analysis indicated that high whole MTV (≥90) and high whole TLG (≥600) were independent predictors of poor PFS and poor OS. In contrast, primary tumor SUV_{max} was not a significant predictor of either PFS or OS. No significant differences were found in FDG parameters for EGFR mutation–negative and EGFR mutation–positive patients.

Posttreatment Metabolic Tumor Volume and Total Lesion Glycolysis are Prognostic

Soussan and colleagues[63] evaluated the prognostic value of volume-based measurements on FDG-PET/CT after induction chemotherapy in 32 patients with stage III NSCLC who were treated with induction platinum-based chemotherapy followed by surgery. The median follow-up time was 19 months (range, 6–43 months). Follow-up (postinduction chemotherapy) SUV_{max}, SUV_{mean}, SUVpeak, TLG, and change in TLG (from baseline to postinduction) of the primary tumor were independent prognostic factors for event-free survival, after adjustment for the effect of surgical treatment, whereas changes in metabolic TLG after induction treatment provided more accurate prognostic information than SUV alone. Separately, Kahraman and colleagues[64] assessed the value of TLG for response prediction and prognostic differentiation in 30 patients with stage IV NSCLC treated with erlotinib. These patients received PET/CT scans before start of therapy, 1 week (early) and 6 weeks (late) after erlotinib treatment. With assessment using different cutoff values for percentage changes of TLG, 20% or 30% change of TLG and lower absolute residual TLG under erlotinib treatment were strong predictive factors for PFS. Winther-Larsen and colleagues[65] also showed that high MTV and TLG were independently correlated with shorter PFS and OS in patients with NSCLC treated with erlotinib.

Volume-Based PET Parameters are Better than Maximum Standardized Uptake Value

Pretreatment metabolic tumor burden, as measured with MTV and TLG, is a prognostic measurement, with a superior correlation to PFS and OS compared with SUV_{max} for NSCLC.[66–68] In 328 surgical and nonsurgical patients with histologically proven NSCLC, the pretreatment whole-body MTV, TLG, whole-body SUV_{max}, and SUV_{mean} of tumors throughout the whole body were measured. SUV_{max}, SUV_{mean}, MTV, and TLG were significantly associated with patients' OS. However, MTV and TLG as metabolic tumor burden measurements were significantly better than SUV_{max} and SUV_{mean}, independent of patients' gender, age, treatment received, TNM stage, whole-body SUV_{max}, and tumor histology.[68]

Multiple studies showed that volume-based PET parameters are significant prognosticators in NSCLC survival even when SUV_{max} or SUV_{mean} of the primary tumor were not.[62,69–72] Hyun and colleagues[72] evaluated the prognostic impact of volume-based assessment by pretreatment FDG-PET/CT in 161 consecutive patients who had stage IIIA-N2 NSCLC treated with neoadjuvant concurrent chemoradiotherapy (CCRT) followed by surgical resection. A higher pretreatment total MTV was significantly associated with poor DFS ($P = .036$) and OS ($P = .012$) in multivariable analysis, which was independent of post-neoadjuvant pathologic stage. In contrast, SUV_{max} of the primary tumor was not significantly associated with DFS and OS. The optimal cutoff total MTV value that allowed risk stratification was 22 cm³: patients with a high total MTV had a significantly shorter median survival time than patients with a low total MTV (median DFS, 11.3 vs 42.0 months, respectively; median OS, 38.3 months vs not reached; $P<.001$ in both

cases). Separately, Zaizen and colleagues[70] retrospectively examined 81 consecutive patients with NSCLC who received chemotherapy and pretreatment FDG-PET. With adjustment for several other variables, Cox regression analysis showed that TLG was significantly prognostic for both PFS (HR = 2.34; $P = .015$) and OS (HR = 2.80; $P = .003$), whereas SUV_{mean} and SUV_{max} were not significantly associated with PFS.

OTHER ^{18}F-fluorodeoxyglucose–PET PARAMETERS
Changes of ^{18}F-Fluorodeoxyglucose Activity as Prognostic Markers

Most studies have been focused on FDG activities at a single-time-point PET scan, either pretreatment or posttreatment. There is evidence that the change of FDG activity from pretreatment to posttreatment FDG-PET also provides important prognostic value in patients with NSCLC.

Han and colleagues[43] evaluated the change in FDG activity as a prognostic factor for early response assessment and survival in patients with NSCLC. The study retrospectively reviewed 33 patients with NSCLC who received first-line chemotherapy. These patients received FDG-PET/CT at initial staging (baseline) and after 2 cycles of chemotherapy (interim PET). The SUV_{max} and MTV of the total malignant lesions were measured in baseline (SUV1 and MTV1) and interim (SUV2 and MTV2) PET images, as well as percentage changes in SUV_{max} (ΔSUV) and MTV (ΔMTV) between baseline and interim PET images. The median follow-up period was 14.3 months with a 2-year OS of 31%. In univariable analysis, in addition to TNM stage, the mean SUV1, MTV1, SUV2, MTV2, ΔSUV, and ΔMTV were all associated significantly with OS. Both the MTV1 and the ΔMTV remained significantly associated with OS in multivariable analyses.[43]

The change in FDG activity in patients with NSCLC was also evaluated as a prognostic factor for tumor recurrence and survival in NSCLC. Huang and colleagues[73] evaluated the value of FDG-PET/CT in predicting recurrence of patients with locally advanced NSCLC during the early stage of CCRT. This prospective study included 53 patients with stage III NSCLC evaluated by FDG-PET before and after radiotherapy with a concurrent cisplatin-based heterogeneous chemotherapy regimen. With a minimum follow-up time of 2 years, these patients had 1-year and 2-year recurrence rates of 18.9% (10 out of 53) and 50.9% (27 out of 53), respectively. Univariate analysis for LRFS revealed 6 variables as having prognostic significance: decrease of SUV_{max} ($P = .007$), intratreatment SUV_{mean} ($P = .029$), decrease of SUV_{mean} ($P = .000$), intratreatment MTV ($P = .006$), decrease of MTV ($P = .000$), and short-term outcome (assessed at 4 weeks after treatment using Response Evaluation Criteria in Solid Tumors [RECIST] criteria) ($P = .000$). Multivariate analysis showed that a decrease in MTV was the only independent prognostic factors for LRFS ($P = .000$; 95% CI, 0.000–0.081). The investigators claimed that the decrease in MTV (using a cutoff of 29.7%) in a primary tumor was the strongest prognostic factor for recurrence for patients with locally advanced NSCLC treated with CCRT. In the same group of patients with NSCLC with CCRT, the investigators also showed that a decrease in MTV (also using a cutoff of 29.7%) in the primary tumor correlated with higher long-term OS.[73] The investigators suggested that tumors with lesser decrease of MTV should be delivered a higher dose of radiation than currently prescribed or changed to other chemotherapy regimens for better tumor control.[71]

Background Activity–Based PET Metrics as Prognostic Markers

Although MTV and TLG have shown promise as prognostic factors for NSCLC, one potential issue is the lack of consensus in choosing the SUV threshold for calculation of these values. Several thresholds from SUV_{max} (40%–50%) as well as absolute thresholds including all voxels with an SUV of 2.5 (TLG2.5) were commonly used for segmentation of tumor sizes.

It was recently shown that a systematic bias exists for PET volume quantification with absolute thresholds or relative thresholds based on SUV_{max}.[74] For example, an adenocarcinoma tumor mass with an SUV_{max} of 2.4 is unmeasurable on MTV or TLG with an absolute threshold of SUV 2.5. In contrast, a lesion with high and uniform FDG activity is likely to be overestimated if a relative threshold of 50% of SUV_{max} is used.

Recent studies have shown that background activity–based PET metrics (background subtracted lesion activity [BSL] and background subtracted volume [BSV]) are promising as prognostic NSCLC markers. BSL is a histogram-based method to determine the tumor activity by subtraction of the background activity from the volume of interest (VOI) surrounding the tumor (using a calculated gaussian fit to the background region to delineate the background activity).

Burger and colleagues[74,75] showed that BSL and BSV were more accurate than TLG in both phantoms and humans.

Burger and colleagues[75] further showed in a study of 44 patients with NSCLC with PET/CT scan before and after neoadjuvant chemotherapy that tumors in good responders after neoadjuvant chemotherapy had significantly lower FDG activity than nonresponding tumors. MTV and TLG based on a 42% fixed threshold for SUV_{max} did not correlate with tumor response, whereas both of the background activity–based PET volume metrics (BSL and BSV) significantly correlated with response ($P<.001$ each). The investigators concluded that PET volume metrics based on background-adaptive methods (BSL and BSV) correlate better with tumor response in patients with NSCLC under neoadjuvant chemotherapy than MTV and TLG using a fixed threshold (42% SUV_{max}).

Steiger and colleagues[76] evaluated 133 patients in early stage I and II NSCLC after surgical resection, and found that volume-based PET metrics do correlate with PFS and OS. These patients had a mean follow-up time of 4.4 years (range, 0.1–10.9 years). Out of 10 potential predictors (histology, stage, volume, SUV_{max}, TLG42%, TLG2.5%, MTV42%, MTV2.5%, BSL, BSV), BSL greater than 6852 ($P = .017$) was chosen as the split point for assigning a patient into a high-risk versus a low-risk group. If BSL was removed from the predictors, TLG42% greater than 4204 ($P = .023$) was chosen as the split point. BSL and TLG42% had similar prognostic performances in this patient group, resulting in nearly the same selections of high-risk patients. The investigators concluded that volume-based PET metrics including total activity (BSL and TLG42%) showed the highest prognostic value among 10 potential predictors.[76]

INCORPORATING QUANTITATIVE PET PARAMETERS INTO NON–SMALL-CELL LUNG CANCER STAGING AND THERAPY RESPONSE CRITERIA

FDG-PET/CT is widely used in patients with lung cancer for staging, restaging, response assessment, and surveillance. SUV_{max} is the most commonly used FDG metric in clinical practice, because it can be obtained easily. It is important in pretreatment and intratreatment that SUV_{max} provides prognostic information before and during treatment, so that therapy strategy can be adjusted accordingly to avoid adverse effects and costs. It makes sense to adjust treatment strategy (eg, chemotherapy dose adjustment, or change to other chemotherapy regimen) based on quantitative FDG changes. MTV and TLG represent three-dimensional measurements incorporating information for both tumor volume and metabolic activity. As a result, MTV/TLG reflects the metabolic status of the entire tumor mass and is more accurate than SUV_{max}, which detects a single-pixel SUV value. Although the maximally active portion of the tumor (SUV_{max} or SUVpeak) may represent the aggressiveness of the tumor, MTV/TLG are more accurate indicators of the overall metabolic status of tumor mass, and thus more accurate prognostic indicators for treatment outcome. It is promising that incorporating metabolic tumor burden information from MTV/TLG may refine risk stratification and predict clinical outcome more accurately in patients with lung cancer.

Although TNM staging remains the major factor in determining treatment outcomes for patients with NSCLC, there is strong evidence corroborating FDG activity as an important prognosticator in lung cancer, from either pretreatment or posttreatment PET scan, regardless of treatment strategy (surgery, radiation or chemotherapy, or a combination of them). The prognostic value of FDG activity is independent of the patient's gender, age, histology, treatment received, as well as the TNM stage.[19,68,77,78] The findings on FDG-PET are used for TNM staging; however, quantitative FDG metrics such as SUV_{max} and MTV/TLG have not been considered in the staging system or in treatment planning.

Compared with other anatomic tumor response metrics, including the World Health Organization (WHO) criteria, the RECIST, and RECIST 1.1, PET-based criteria such as EORTC (European Organization for Research and Treatment of Cancer) and PERCIST (PET Response Criteria in Solid Tumors)[79] have the advantages of incorporating tumor metabolic activity in evaluating tumor response, because change in tumor size can be minimal and late despite effective treatment, making anatomy-based response criteria less effective. Multiple studies have shown that PERCIST outperforms RECIST in the evaluation of tumor response to treatment[80,81] and has been associated with statistically significant differences in survival in patients with NSCLC[82,83] and SCLC.[84] In a group of 44 patients with NSCLC treated by chemotherapy, Ding and colleagues[82] showed that PERCIST, but not RECIST, was a significant factor for predicting DFS (HR, 3.20; 95% CI, 1.85–5.54; $P<.001$). However, the volumetric changes in FDG activity or FDG-avid tumor load are not an integrated part of the current PET

response criteria. The EORTC recommends mean and maximum SUVs corrected for body surface area, whereas PERCIST recommends the SUV_{peak} corrected for lean body mass.

Both EORTC and PERCIST criteria recommend using quantitative changes in SUV as indications of therapy response in solid tumors. For example, EORTC recommends a reduction of at least 25% in SUV_{mean} (normalized body surface area), whereas PERCIST advises a reduction of at least 30% in SUV_{peak} (normalized to lean body mass) and an absolute decrease of 0.8 SUV units as a criterion for partial metabolic response to treatment. However, the absolute value of SUVs and volume-based PET parameters are not considered.

The findings of MTV/TLG in multiple studies as an important prognostic factor for patients with NSCLC, with better value than that of SUV_{max}, SUV_{mean}, and SUV_{peak}, are clinically very important. There are limited studies in the literature evaluating the association between SUV_{peak} and prognosis, and very few on lung cancer. The authors noted that the prospective ACRIN 6668/Radiation Therapy Oncology Group 0235 trial showed that the independent prognostic value of pretreatment MTV in patients with inoperable stage III NSCLC was from SUV_{peak} (as well as performance status, stage, age, gender).[61] A retrospective review of prospectively collected data from 23 patients with metastatic lung adenocarcinoma treated with erlotinib revealed that systemic TLG criteria were superior to both EORTC and PERCIST for predicting outcomes of 2-year PFS and OS, using SUV greater than 2.5 as the threshold for target volume delineation of the MTV. Patients who were classified as responders on day 14 based on TLG criteria had higher 2-year PFS (26.7% vs 0%; $P = .007$; HR = 0.28; 95% CI = 0.10–0.76; $P = .012$), and higher 2-year OS (40.0% vs 7.7%; $P = .018$; HR = 0.32; 95% CI = 0.12–0.86; $P = .024$). In contrast, the assessment of early response based on PERCIST criteria was not significantly associated with PFS or OS.[85] It was also reported that the use of SUV_{peak} for assessment of treatment response can be significantly affected by subjective issues, because the definition of ROI (the size, shape, and location of ROI) resulted in substantial variation ($\geq$50%) in both SUV_{peak} and tumor response for individual tumors.[86] However, data are limited in the literature regarding comparison of MTV/TLG versus available therapy response criteria such as PERCIST. Future studies are needed to confirm the findings.

HINDRANCES THAT LIMIT CLINICAL USE OF QUANTITATIVE PET PARAMETERS

Several questions remain to be answered before the SUV_{max} (or SUV_{peak}) and volume-based FDG parameters can be included in the prognosis assessment of lung cancer, either during initial staging or for intratreatment response evaluation.

It is easy to note that there is a wide SUV value cutoff range in the primary tumor to discriminate between a favorable and unfavorable prognosis in patients with NSCLC. The SUV_{max} cutoff ranged from 5 to 15 in a meta-analysis of prognostic significance of SUV_{max} in NSCLC treated with radiotherapy.[87] The SUV_{max} cutoff ranged from 2.4 to 20 in a meta-analysis of prognostic significance of pretreatment SUV_{max} in surgically treated NSCLC.[59] The wide range of SUV cutoff values could be caused by technical issues, tumor heterogeneity, or variation of the patient cohorts analyzed. Methods used to determine the SUV_{max} cutoff threshold also vary, with the optimal cutoff value and the median SUV_{max} value being most frequently used, and a few studies used SUV_{max} of 2.5 and an arbitrary value as a cutoff.[58] Noted that these optimal PET parameter cutoffs that best discriminated the survival curves in each study may apply to that specific patient population only, and cannot be generalized to clinical practice.

The lack of consensus regarding an optimal SUV_{max} cutoff value significantly limits its clinical application, and such a consensus value may be hard to define in the near future. In a study of 498 patients with primary lung cancer reported by Davies and colleagues,[88] there was continuous worsening in survival with increasing SUV_{max}, consistently observed at 12 months, 18 months, and 24 months. Clarke and colleagues[39] also showed that, when pretreatment SUV_{max} was assessed as a continuous variable, there was continued increase in HR regarding regional relapse and distant metastasis with each unit increase in pre-SBRT SUV_{max} in patients with medically inoperable early-stage NSCLC (although SUV_{max} 5 was the optimal cutoff value). Downey and colleagues[22] showed that, in patients with NSCLC (T1–T4, N0–N2, M0) treated by R0 resection, each unit of pretreatment SUV_{max} increase corresponded with a 7% increase in the risk of death. In addition, it has been reported that the SUV_{max}, SUV70%, and SUV50% hold a similar prognostic value in resectable NSCLC.[89] These findings may indicate that FDG activity is only one of many factors affecting prognosis, and the relationship between SUV and prognosis is a gradual and proportional phenomenon rather than a threshold-based effect, with a continuous increase in the hazard as SUV increases.

As with SUV_{max}, various thresholding methods have been applied to volume-based PET analyses, and an optimal threshold has not yet been established. The reported cutoff ranges from 0.3 to 68.3 cm^3 for MTV and from 9.6 to 525 for TLG in patients with NSCLC.[90] Also, similarly to SUV_{max}, there is evidence of continuous worsening of lung cancer prognosis in response to further increases of MTV or TLG. The prospective ACRIN 6668/Radiation Therapy Oncology Group 0235 trial showed that every 10-cm^3 increase in pretreatment MTV was associated with a 3% increase in risk of death ($P<.001$), after controlling for other variables.[61] It is possible that, as with SUV_{max}, the FDG-avid tumor burden (as represented by MTV and TLG) may have a gradual and proportional prognostic effect in NSCLC without a definite cutoff value.

In addition, there are unique obstacles when dealing with MTV/TLG. Although SUV_{max} is easy to obtain, readily available, and shows no interobserver variability, the opposite is true for MTV/TLG. The measurement of MTV or TLG is time consuming, is not available with standard PET/CT software (it requires a special software/workstation for calculation), and is not a standard clinical practice at this time. More important, the calculation for MTV/TLG is subjective and depends on how the threshold SUV is selected, a method that varies significantly in the literature. For MTV segmentation, various thresholds of SUV activity have been used, including absolute threshold of SUV of 2.5, or using relative thresholds of either 40% or 50% of the maximum intratumoral FDG activity, with the most commonly used threshold of 42% of SUV_{max}. The resulting MTV and TLG values vary significantly, depending on the threshold selected.[90]

However, it is possible that the prognostic value of MTV/TLG may exist regardless of the SUV threshold selected. Kim and colleagues[91] evaluated the usefulness of the preoperative FDG-avid tumor burden in predicting RFS and OS in surgically resected patients with NSCLC. The study included 91 patients with pathologically documented stages I to IIIA NSCLC. Preoperative MTV and TLG were obtained with thresholds of SUV 2.5, 3.0, 3.5, and 4.0. Patients with smaller MTVs and lower TLGs had a better OS, irrespective of the SUV thresholds selected for the calculation of MTV or TLG, and no significant association was found between the type of operation and volumetric parameters.

SUMMARY

Personalized medicine is a major focus in modern cancer therapy and is intended to provide optimal treatment of individual patients based on tumor characteristics and TNM staging. This approach takes into consideration the presentation of clinical features, imaging features, pathologic findings, and patient-specific and tumor-specific biology and genomics, so that a personalized treatment can be provided for an expected patient-specific outcome. FDG-avid tumor load parameters, including SUV_{max} but better represented by MTV and TLG, seem to be promising tumor prognostic indicators in NSCLC. The ability to predict tumor behavior in treatment before therapy begins, as well as the capacity to assess tumor response to each stage of treatment, are among the most important factors in successful personalized cancer treatment. The incorporation of quantitative FDG activity in tumor staging and therapy response criteria in the future, despite requiring further validation, is likely to allow better risk stratification so that better treatment outcomes can be reached while avoiding unnecessary treatment procedures, side effects, and costs. Further large-scale, prospective investigations of the role of FDG-PET in lung cancer prognosis are warranted to determine more accurate prognostic significance and optimal cutoff values.

REFERENCES

1. American Cancer Society. Key statistics for lung cancer. 2016. Available at: http://www.cancer.org/cancer/lungcancer-non-smallcell/detailedguide/non-small-cell-lung-cancer-key-statistics. Accessed July 9, 2016.
2. Curran WJ Jr, Paulus R, Langer CJ, et al. Sequential vs. concurrent chemoradiation for stage III non-small cell lung cancer: randomized phase III trial RTOG 9410. J Natl Cancer Inst 2011;103(19):1452–60.
3. Ginsberg MS, Grewal RK, Heelan RT. Lung cancer. Radiol Clin North Am 2007;45(1):21–43.
4. Podoloff DA, Advani RH, Allred C, et al. NCCN task force report: positron emission tomography (PET)/computed tomography (CT) scanning in cancer. J Natl Compr Cancer Netw 2007;5(Suppl 1):S1–22 [quiz: S23-2].
5. Ruilong Z, Daohai X, Li G, et al. Diagnostic value of 18F-FDG-PET/CT for the evaluation of solitary pulmonary nodules: a systematic review and meta-analysis. Nucl Med Commun 2017;38(1):67–75.
6. Ung YC, Maziak DE, Vanderveen JA, et al. 18Fluorodeoxyglucose positron emission tomography in the diagnosis and staging of lung cancer: a systematic review. J Natl Cancer Inst 2007;99(23):1753–67.
7. Huellner MW, de Galiza Barbosa F, Husmann L, et al. TNM staging of non-small cell lung cancer: comparison of PET/MR and PET/CT. J Nucl Med 2016;57(1):21–6.
8. Hicks RJ. Role of 18F-FDG PET in assessment of response in non-small cell lung cancer. J Nucl Med 2009;50(Suppl 1):31S–42S.
9. Onishi Y, Ohno Y, Koyama H, et al. Non-small cell carcinoma: comparison of postoperative intra- and extrathoracic recurrence assessment capability of qualitatively and/or quantitatively assessed FDG-PET/CT and standard radiological examinations. Eur J Radiol 2011;79(3):473–9.
10. van den Berg LL, Klinkenberg TJ, Groen HJM, et al. Patterns of recurrence and survival after surgery or stereotactic radiotherapy for early stage NSCLC. J Thorac Oncol 2015;10(5):826–31.
11. Sheikhbahaei S, Mena E, Yanamadala A, et al. The value of FDG PET/CT in treatment response assessment, follow-up, and surveillance of lung cancer. AJR Am J Roentgenol 2017;208(2):420–33.
12. van Rens MT, de la Riviere AB, Elbers HR, et al. Prognostic assessment of 2,361 patients who underwent pulmonary resection for non-small cell lung cancer, stage I, II, and IIIA. Chest 2000;117(2):374–9.
13. Choi N, Baumann M, Flentjie M, et al. Predictive factors in radiotherapy for non-small cell lung cancer: present status. Lung Cancer 2001;31(1):43–56.
14. Borst GR, Belderbos JSA, Boellaard R, et al. Standardised FDG uptake: a prognostic factor for inoperable non-small cell lung cancer. Eur J Cancer 2005;41(11):1533–41.
15. Arslan D, Bozcuk H, Gunduz S, et al. Survival results and prognostic factors in T4 N0-3 non-small cell lung cancer patients according to the AJCC 7th edition staging system. Asian Pac J Cancer Prev 2014;15(6):2465–72.
16. Horne ZD, Clump DA, Vargo JA, et al. Pretreatment SUVmax predicts progression-free survival in early-stage non-small cell lung cancer treated with stereotactic body radiation therapy. Radiat Oncol 2014;9:41.
17. Kohutek ZA, Wu AJ, Zhang Z, et al. FDG-PET maximum standardized uptake value is prognostic for recurrence and survival after stereotactic body radiotherapy for non-small cell lung cancer. Lung Cancer 2015;89(2):115–20.
18. Stanley KE. Prognostic factors for survival in patients with inoperable lung cancer. J Natl Cancer Inst 1980;65(1):25–32.
19. Um S-W, Kim H, Koh W-J, et al. Prognostic value of 18F-FDG uptake on positron emission tomography in patients with pathologic stage I non-small cell lung cancer. J Thorac Oncol 2009;4(11):1331–6.

20. Ordu C, Selcuk NA, Erdogan E, et al. Does early PET/CT assesment of response to chemotherapy predicts survival in patients with advanced stage non-small-cell lung cancer? Medicine 2014; 93(28):e299.
21. Filderman AE, Silvestri GA, Gatsonis C, et al. Prognostic significance of tumor proliferative fraction and DNA content in stage I non-small cell lung cancer. Am Rev Respir Dis 1992;146(3):707–10.
22. Downey RJ, Akhurst T, Gonen M, et al. Preoperative F-18 fluorodeoxyglucose-positron emission tomography maximal standardized uptake value predicts survival after lung cancer resection. J Clin Oncol 2004;22(16):3255–60.
23. Tang H, Wang S, Xiao G, et al. Comprehensive evaluation of published gene expression prognostic signatures for biomarker-based lung cancer clinical studies. Ann Oncol 2017;28(4):733–40.
24. Jeong HJ, Min JJ, Park JM, et al. Determination of the prognostic value of [(18)F]fluorodeoxyglucose uptake by using positron emission tomography in patients with non-small cell lung cancer. Nucl Med Commun 2002;23(9):865–70.
25. Sasaki R, Komaki R, Macapinlac H, et al. [18F]fluorodeoxyglucose uptake by positron emission tomography predicts outcome of non-small-cell lung cancer. J Clin Oncol 2005;23(6):1136–43.
26. Cerfolio RJ, Bryant AS, Ohja B, et al. The maximum standardized uptake values on positron emission tomography of a non-small cell lung cancer predict stage, recurrence, and survival. J Thorac Cardiovasc Surg 2005;130(1):151–9.
27. Eschmann SM, Friedel G, Paulsen F, et al. Is standardised (18)F-FDG uptake value an outcome predictor in patients with stage III non-small cell lung cancer? Eur J Nucl Med Mol Imaging 2006;33(3):263–9 [Erratum appears in Eur J Nucl Med Mol Imaging 2006;33(3):389].
28. Mac Manus MP, Hicks RJ, Matthews JP, et al. Positron emission tomography is superior to computed tomography scanning for response-assessment after radical radiotherapy or chemoradiotherapy in patients with non-small-cell lung cancer. J Clin Oncol 2003;21(7):1285–92.
29. Hellwig D, Graeter TP, Ukena D, et al. Value of F-18-fluorodeoxyglucose positron emission tomography after induction therapy of locally advanced bronchogenic carcinoma. J Thorac Cardiovasc Surg 2004; 128(6):892–9.
30. Hoekstra CJ, Stroobants SG, Smit EF, et al. Prognostic relevance of response evaluation using [18F]-2-fluoro-2-deoxy-D-glucose positron emission tomography in patients with locally advanced non-small-cell lung cancer. J Clin Oncol 2005;23(33): 8362–70.
31. Hicks RJ, Kalff V, MacManus MP, et al. The utility of (18)F-FDG PET for suspected recurrent non-small cell lung cancer after potentially curative therapy: impact on management and prognostic stratification. J Nucl Med 2001;42(11):1605–13.
32. Hellwig D, Groschel A, Graeter TP, et al. Diagnostic performance and prognostic impact of FDG-PET in suspected recurrence of surgically treated non-small cell lung cancer. Eur J Nucl Med Mol Imaging 2006;33(1):13–21.
33. Murakami S, Saito H, Sakuma Y, et al. Prognostic value of preoperative FDG-PET in stage IA lung adenocarcinoma. Eur J Radiol 2012;81(8):1891–5.
34. Goodgame B, Pillot GA, Yang Z, et al. Prognostic value of preoperative positron emission tomography in resected stage I non-small cell lung cancer. J Thorac Oncol 2008;3(2):130–4.
35. Higuchi M, Hasegawa T, Osugi J, et al. Prognostic impact of FDG-PET in surgically treated pathological stage I lung adenocarcinoma. Ann Thorac Cardiovasc Surg 2014;20(3):185–91.
36. Konings R, van Gool MH, Bard MPL, et al. Prognostic value of pre-operative glucose-corrected maximum standardized uptake value in patients with non-small cell lung cancer after complete surgical resection and 5-year follow-up. Ann Nucl Med 2016;30(5):362–8.
37. Hamamoto Y, Sugawara Y, Inoue T, et al. Relationship between pretreatment FDG uptake and local control after stereotactic body radiotherapy in stage I non-small-cell lung cancer: the preliminary results. Jpn J Clin Oncol 2011;41(4):543–7.
38. Takeda A, Yokosuka N, Ohashi T, et al. The maximum standardized uptake value (SUVmax) on FDG-PET is a strong predictor of local recurrence for localized non-small-cell lung cancer after stereotactic body radiotherapy (SBRT). Radiother Oncol 2011;101(2):291–7.
39. Clarke K, Taremi M, Dahele M, et al. Stereotactic body radiotherapy (SBRT) for non-small cell lung cancer (NSCLC): is FDG-PET a predictor of outcome? Radiother Oncol 2012;104(1):62–6.
40. Imamura Y, Azuma K, Kurata S, et al. Prognostic value of SUVmax measurements obtained by FDG-PET in patients with non-small cell lung cancer receiving chemotherapy. Lung Cancer 2011;71(1): 49–54.
41. Dooms C, Verbeken E, Stroobants S, et al. Prognostic stratification of stage IIIA-N2 non-small-cell lung cancer after induction chemotherapy: a model based on the combination of morphometric-pathologic response in mediastinal nodes and primary tumor response on serial 18-fluoro-2-deoxy-glucose positron emission tomography. J Clin Oncol 2008;26(7):1128–34.
42. Decoster L, Schallier D, Everaert H, et al. Complete metabolic tumour response, assessed by 18-fluorodeoxyglucose positron emission tomography (18FDG-PET), after induction chemotherapy predicts

a favourable outcome in patients with locally advanced non-small cell lung cancer (NSCLC). Lung Cancer 2008;62(1):55–61.

43. Han EJ, Yang YJ, Park JC, et al. Prognostic value of early response assessment using 18F-FDG PET/CT in chemotherapy-treated patients with non-small-cell lung cancer. Nucl Med Commun 2015;36(12):1187–94.

44. Kim SH, Lee JH, Lee GJ, et al. Interpretation and prognostic value of positron emission tomography-computed tomography after induction chemotherapy with or without radiation in IIIA-N2 non-small cell lung cancer patients who receive curative surgery. Medicine 2015;94(24):e955.

45. Ripley RT, Suzuki K, Tan KS, et al. Postinduction positron emission tomography assessment of N2 nodes is not associated with ypN2 disease or overall survival in stage IIIA non-small cell lung cancer. J Thorac Cardiovasc Surg 2016;151(4):969–77.

46. Barnett SA, Downey RJ, Zheng J, et al. Utility of routine PET imaging to predict response and survival after induction therapy for non-small cell lung cancer. Ann Thorac Surg 2016;101(3):1052–9.

47. Kamel MK, Rahouma M, Ghaly G, et al. Clinical predictors of persistent mediastinal nodal disease after induction therapy for stage IIIA N2 non-small cell lung cancer. Ann Thorac Surg 2017;103(1):281–6.

48. Tanvetyanon T, Eikman EA, Sommers E, et al. Computed tomography response, but not positron emission tomography scan response, predicts survival after neoadjuvant chemotherapy for resectable non-small-cell lung cancer. J Clin Oncol 2008;26(28):4610–6.

49. Skoura E, Datseris IE, Platis I, et al. Role of positron emission tomography in the early prediction of response to chemotherapy in patients with non–small-cell lung cancer. Clin Lung Cancer 2012;13(3):181–7.

50. Xiang Z-L, Erasmus J, Komaki R, et al. FDG uptake correlates with recurrence and survival after treatment of unresectable stage III non-small cell lung cancer with high-dose proton therapy and chemotherapy. Radiat Oncol 2012;7:144.

51. Machtay M, Duan F, Siegel BA, et al. Prediction of survival by [18F]fluorodeoxyglucose positron emission tomography in patients with locally advanced non-small-cell lung cancer undergoing definitive chemoradiation therapy: results of the ACRIN 6668/RTOG 0235 trial. J Clin Oncol 2013;31(30):3823–30.

52. Ikushima H, Dong L, Erasmus J, et al. Predictive value of 18F-fluorodeoxyglucose uptake by positron emission tomography for non-small cell lung cancer patients treated with radical radiotherapy. J Radiat Res 2010;51(4):465–71.

53. Ryu JS, Choi NC, Fischman AJ, et al. FDG-PET in staging and restaging non-small cell lung cancer after neoadjuvant chemoradiotherapy: correlation with histopathology. Lung Cancer 2002;35(2):179–87.

54. Hoopes DJ, Tann M, Fletcher JW, et al. FDG-PET and stereotactic body radiotherapy (SBRT) for stage I non-small-cell lung cancer. Lung Cancer 2007;56(2):229–34.

55. Burdick MJ, Stephans KL, Reddy CA, et al. Maximum standardized uptake value from staging FDG-PET/CT does not predict treatment outcome for early-stage non-small-cell lung cancer treated with stereotactic body radiotherapy. Int J Radiat Oncol Biol Phys 2010;78(4):1033–9.

56. Win T, Miles KA, Janes SM, et al. Tumor heterogeneity and permeability as measured on the CT component of PET/CT predict survival in patients with non-small cell lung cancer. Clin Cancer Res 2013;19(13):3591–9.

57. Vesselle H, Freeman JD, Wiens L, et al. Fluorodeoxyglucose uptake of primary non-small cell lung cancer at positron emission tomography: new contrary data on prognostic role. Clin Cancer Res 2007;13(11):3255–63.

58. Paesmans M, Berghmans T, Dusart M, et al. Primary tumor standardized uptake value measured on fluorodeoxyglucose positron emission tomography is of prognostic value for survival in non-small cell lung cancer: update of a systematic review and meta-analysis by the European Lung Cancer Working Party for the International Association for the Study of Lung Cancer Staging Project. J Thorac Oncol 2010;5(5):612–9.

59. Liu J, Dong M, Sun X, et al. Prognostic value of 18F-FDG PET/CT in surgical non-small cell lung cancer: a meta-analysis. PLoS One 2016;11(1):e0146195.

60. Dong M, Liu J, Sun X, et al. Prognostic significance of SUVmax on pretreatment 18 F-FDG PET/CT in early-stage non-small cell lung cancer treated with stereotactic body radiotherapy: a meta-analysis. J Med Imaging Radiat Oncol 2017. [Epub ahead of print].

61. Bazan JG, Duan F, Snyder BS, et al. Metabolic tumor volume predicts overall survival and local control in patients with stage III non-small cell lung cancer treated in ACRIN 6668/RTOG 0235. Eur J Nucl Med Mol Imaging 2017;44(1):17–24.

62. Chung HW, Lee KY, Kim HJ, et al. FDG PET/CT metabolic tumor volume and total lesion glycolysis predict prognosis in patients with advanced lung adenocarcinoma. J Cancer Res Clin Oncol 2014;140(1):89–98.

63. Soussan M, Chouahnia K, Maisonobe J-A, et al. Prognostic implications of volume-based measurements on FDG PET/CT in stage III non-small-cell lung cancer after induction chemotherapy. Eur J Nucl Med Mol Imaging 2013;40(5):668–76.

64. Kahraman D, Holstein A, Scheffler M, et al. Tumor lesion glycolysis and tumor lesion proliferation for response prediction and prognostic differentiation in patients with advanced non-small cell lung cancer treated with erlotinib. Clin Nucl Med 2012;37(11):1058–64.

65. Winther-Larsen A, Fledelius J, Sorensen BS, et al. Metabolic tumor burden as marker of outcome in advanced EGFR wild-type NSCLC patients treated with erlotinib. Lung Cancer 2016;94:81–7.

66. Liao S, Penney BC, Zhang H, et al. Prognostic value of the quantitative metabolic volumetric measurement on 18F-FDG PET/CT in stage IV nonsurgical small-cell lung cancer. Acad Radiol 2012;19(1):69–77.

67. Chen HHW, Chiu N-T, Su W-C, et al. Prognostic value of whole-body total lesion glycolysis at pretreatment FDG PET/CT in non-small cell lung cancer. Radiology 2012;264(2):559–66.

68. Zhang H, Wroblewski K, Appelbaum D, et al. Independent prognostic value of whole-body metabolic tumor burden from FDG-PET in non-small cell lung cancer. Int J Comput Assist Radiol Surg 2013;8(2):181–91.

69. Yan H, Wang R, Zhao F, et al. Measurement of tumor volume by PET to evaluate prognosis in patients with advanced non-small cell lung cancer treated by non-surgical therapy. Acta Radiol 2011;52(6):646–50 [Retraction in Skjennald A. Acta Radiol 2012;53(6):592].

70. Zaizen Y, Azuma K, Kurata S, et al. Prognostic significance of total lesion glycolysis in patients with advanced non-small cell lung cancer receiving chemotherapy. Eur J Radiol 2012;81(12):4179–84.

71. Huang W, Liu B, Fan M, et al. The early predictive value of a decrease of metabolic tumor volume in repeated (18)F-FDG PET/CT for recurrence of locally advanced non-small cell lung cancer with concurrent radiochemotherapy. Eur J Radiol 2015;84(3):482–8.

72. Hyun SH, Ahn HK, Ahn M-J, et al. Volume-based assessment with 18F-FDG PET/CT improves outcome prediction for patients with stage IIIA-N2 non-small cell lung cancer. AJR Am J Roentgenol 2015;205(3):623–8.

73. Huang W, Fan M, Liu B, et al. Value of metabolic tumor volume on repeated 18F-FDG PET/CT for early prediction of survival in locally advanced non-small cell lung cancer treated with concurrent chemoradiotherapy. J Nucl Med 2014;55(10):1584–90.

74. Burger IA, Vargas HA, Apte A, et al. PET quantification with a histogram derived total activity metric: superior quantitative consistency compared to total lesion glycolysis with absolute or relative SUV thresholds in phantoms and lung cancer patients. Nucl Med Biol 2014;41(5):410–8.

75. Burger IA, Casanova R, Steiger S, et al. 18F-FDG PET/CT of non-small cell lung carcinoma under neoadjuvant chemotherapy: background-based adaptive-volume metrics outperform TLG and MTV in predicting histopathologic response. J Nucl Med 2016;57(6):849–54.

76. Steiger S, Arvanitakis M, Sick B, et al. Analysis of prognostic values of various PET metrics in preoperative FDG PET for early stage bronchial carcinoma for progression free and overall survival: significantly increased glycolysis is a predictive factor. J Nucl Med 2017. [Epub ahead of print].

77. Hanin F-X, Lonneux M, Cornet J, et al. Prognostic value of FDG uptake in early stage non-small cell lung cancer. Eur J Cardiothorac Surg 2008;33(5):819–23.

78. Nair VS, Barnett PG, Ananth L, et al. PET scan 18F-fluorodeoxyglucose uptake and prognosis in patients with resected clinical stage IA non-small cell lung cancer. Chest 2010;137(5):1150–6.

79. Wahl RL, Jacene H, Kasamon Y, et al. From RECIST to PERCIST: evolving considerations for PET response criteria in solid tumors. J Nucl Med 2009;50(Suppl 1):122S–50S.

80. Min SJ, Jang HJ, Kim JH. Comparison of the RECIST and PERCIST criteria in solid tumors: a pooled analysis and review. Oncotarget 2016;7(19):27848–54.

81. Shang J, Ling X, Zhang L, et al. Comparison of RECIST, EORTC criteria and PERCIST for evaluation of early response to chemotherapy in patients with non-small-cell lung cancer. Eur J Nucl Med Mol Imaging 2016;43(11):1945–53.

82. Ding Q, Cheng X, Yang L, et al. PET/CT evaluation of response to chemotherapy in non-small cell lung cancer: PET response criteria in solid tumors (PERCIST) versus response evaluation criteria in solid tumors (RECIST). J Thorac Dis 2014;6(6):677–83.

83. Fledelius J, Khalil AA, Hjorthaug K, et al. Using positron emission tomography (PET) response criteria in solid tumours (PERCIST) 1.0 for evaluation of 2'-deoxy-2'-[18F] fluoro-D-glucose-PET/CT scans to predict survival early during treatment of locally advanced non-small cell lung cancer (NSCLC). J Med Imaging Radiat Oncol 2016;60(2):231–8.

84. Ziai D, Wagner T, El Badaoui A, et al. Therapy response evaluation with FDG-PET/CT in small cell lung cancer: a prognostic and comparison study of the PERCIST and EORTC criteria. Cancer Imaging 2013;13:73–80.

85. Ho K-C, Fang Y-HD, Chung H-W, et al. TLG-S criteria are superior to both EORTC and PERCIST for predicting outcomes in patients with metastatic lung adenocarcinoma treated with erlotinib. Eur J Nucl Med Mol Imaging 2016;43(12):2155–65.

86. Vanderhoek M, Perlman SB, Jeraj R. Impact of the definition of peak standardized uptake value on quantification of treatment response. J Nucl Med 2012;53(1):4–11.

87. Na F, Wang J, Li C, et al. Primary tumor standardized uptake value measured on F18-Fluorodeoxyglucose positron emission tomography is of prediction value for survival and local control in non-small-cell lung cancer receiving radiotherapy: meta-analysis. J Thorac Oncol 2014;9(6):834–42.

88. Davies A, Tan C, Paschalides C, et al. FDG-PET maximum standardised uptake value is associated with variation in survival: analysis of 498 lung cancer patients. Lung Cancer 2007;55(1):75–8.

89. de Jong WK, van der Heijden HFM, Pruim J, et al. Prognostic value of different metabolic measurements with fluorine-18 fluorodeoxyglucose positron emission tomography in resectable non-small cell lung cancer: a two-center study. J Thorac Oncol 2007;2(11):1007–12.

90. Im H-J, Pak K, Cheon GJ, et al. Prognostic value of volumetric parameters of (18)F-FDG PET in non-small-cell lung cancer: a meta-analysis. Eur J Nucl Med Mol Imaging 2015;42(2):241–51.

91. Kim K, Kim S-J, Kim I-J, et al. Prognostic value of volumetric parameters measured by F-18 FDG PET/CT in surgically resected non-small-cell lung cancer. Nucl Med Commun 2012;33(6):613–20.

Non–Small-Cell Lung Cancer PET Imaging Beyond F18 Fluorodeoxyglucose

Gang Cheng, MD, PhD

KEYWORDS

• Lung cancer • PET/CT • Carcinoid • Proliferation • Hypoxia • Angiogenesis • Personalized therapy

KEY POINTS

- Non–small-cell lung cancer (NSCLC) has significant heterogeneity histologically, biologically, and molecularly.
- F18 Fluorodeoxyglucose (FDG) is a nonspecific PET tracer. Although useful, FDG PET is not able to define the entire complexity of NSCLC heterogeneity.
- Gallium-68 (^{68}Ga)-somatostatin analog PET imaging has significantly improved diagnosis of well-differentiated pulmonary carcinoid tumors.
- PET tracers targeting tumor proliferation, hypoxia, and angiogenesis are promising for improving the sensitivity and specificity of PET imaging for better lesion characterization, treatment stratification, and therapeutic monitoring.
- PET tracers designed to characterize driver genes and pathway-specific targets could provide noninvasive key information in tumor genetic characterization for personalized therapy in NSCLC patients.

INTRODUCTION

F18 Fluorodeoxyglucose (FDG) PET/CT is now widely used clinically and has revolutionized tumor staging, restaging, treatment planning, and prognosis assessment in lung cancer and many other malignancies. The interpretation of FDG PET is dependent, however, on tissue glucose metabolism, which is not malignancy specific. Not all malignancies are FDG avid. Many benign etiologies, especially inflammatory/infectious changes, may cause increased FDG activity. It is not rare to have false-positive and false-negative findings on an FDG PET scan.[1,2] Furthermore, all histologic subtypes of lung cancer have significant heterogeneity—histologically, biologically, and molecularly.[3] In addition to energy metabolism, multiple microenvironmental factors, including hypoxia

and angiogenesis, may affect tumor progression and treatment response. Tumor heterogeneity may present in different tumor masses within the same person, and even within the same tumor mass. The presence of significant tumor heterogeneity may affect treatment outcome. FDG PET, although useful, is not able to define the entire complexity of NSCLC heterogeneity. As a result, more specific PET imaging probes are extremely valuable for accurate tumor staging studies and to determine response to treatment.

Traditionally, histologic findings serve as the most important findings guiding treatment decisions in non–small-cell lung cancer (NSCLC) and other malignancies. This has changed significantly in the past decade, because molecular diagnostics may provide critical information of driver mutations in lung cancer patients to help selecting the best

Disclosure Statement: None.
Department of Radiology, Hospital of the University of Pennsylvania, 3400 Spruce Street, Philadelphia, PA 19104, USA
E-mail address: gang.cheng@uphs.upenn.edu

targeted agent for personalized patient care. NSCLC subtypes are divided not only by histology criteria but also by molecular characteristics. Many oncogene mutations, such as epidermal growth factor receptor (EGFR) and anaplastic lymphoma kinase (ALK), have been identified as important tumor markers and critical targets in NSCLC therapy. Much progress has been made recently for lung cancer in recent years to develop new PET tracers to improve the sensitivity and specificity of PET imaging for better lesion characterization, treatment stratification, and therapeutic monitoring. Especially, recent development in molecular diagnostics and targeting agents for genomically defined lung cancer patients have brought in a new era in the diagnosis and treatment of lung cancer. Although most of these new tracers are in the early stages of development or are still under research, they represent the future of PET imaging with unlimited potential clinical value. This article reviews some of current progresses of PET imaging other than FDG in development, clinical practice, and potential future applications.

TRACERS IN PULMONARY NEUROENDOCRINE TUMORS

Pulmonary neuroendocrine tumors are a heterogeneous group of malignancies that arise from neuroendocrine cells (Kulchitsky cells), including low-grade (typical carcinoid), intermediate-grade (atypical carcinoid), and high-grade malignancies (large cell neuroendocrine carcinoma and small cell lung cancer).[4,5] High-grade pulmonary neuroendocrine tumors tend to have high FDG activity. A well-differentiated typical carcinoid (accounting for 2% of primary lung neoplasms), however, often with intense enhancement in contrast-enhanced CT study, generally has low uptake on FDG PET/CT imaging, (see Yiyan Liu's article, "Lung Neoplasms with Low F18-Fluorodeoxyglucose Avidity," in this issue).

The development of ^{68}Ga-1,4,7,10-tetraazacyclododecane-N,N′,N″,N‴-tetraacetic acid-d-Phe1,Tyr3-octreotate (^{68}Ga-DOTATATE) (Food and Drug Administration approved) and other somatostatin-based PET tracers (^{68}Ga-DOTATOC and ^{68}Ga-DOTANOC) have significantly improved diagnosis of neuroendocrine tumors including pulmonary carcinoid. All 3 (DOTATOC, DOTANOC, and DOTATATE) PET tracers bind specifically to subtypes 2 of somatostatin receptor (SSTR). DOTANOC also presents a good affinity for subtypes 2, 3, and 5 of SSTR. ^{68}Ga–DOTA-peptides PET imaging offers multiple advantages over traditional SSTR scintigraphy (indium ^{111}In–pentetreotide), including a much higher affinity for SSTRs,

superior resolution and contrast, and shorter examination times, making it superior to ^{111}In–DTPA-pentetreotide single-photon emission CT (SPECT) or SPECT/CT imaging in the diagnosis of pulmonary and gastroenteropancreatic neuroendocrine tumors.[6]

For patients with suspected pulmonary carcinoid tumors, somatostatin-based PET significantly outperformed FDG PET. Venkitaraman and colleagues[7] performed a prospective study, including 32 patients with clinical suspicion of bronchopulmonary carcinoid. These patients were evaluated with ^{68}Ga-DOTATOC PET/CT and FDG PET/CT. Using tissue diagnosis as the reference standard (confirmed 21 typical carcinoid tumors, 5 atypical carcinoids, and 6 noncarcinoid tumors), the sensitivity, specificity, and accuracy of ^{68}Ga-DOTATOC PET/CT in the diagnosis of pulmonary carcinoid tumor were 96.15, 100%, and 96.87%, respectively, whereas those of FDG PET/CT were 78.26, 11.1% and 59.37%, respectively. More recently, Walker and colleagues[8] also demonstrated that ^{68}Ga-DOTATATE PET is more specific than FDG PET in the evaluation of indeterminate pulmonary nodules.

Incorporating ^{111}In–DTPA-octreotide[9] or ^{68}Ga-DOTATATE[10] ^{68}Ga-DOTATOC[11,12] imaging to FDG PET could improve sensitivity and specificity in the diagnosis of pulmonary carcinoid tumors. Indolent tumors, such as typical well-differentiated bronchial carcinoids, have low FDG uptake (therefore, FDG PET is of limited use at discriminating tumors from scars and distal atelectasis in these patients) but have high uptake on ^{68}Ga-DOTATATE PET imaging (which makes differential diagnosis easy and simple), whereas atypical and higher-grade carcinoids have less ^{68}Ga-DOTATATE avidity but are more FDG avid.[10] There is strong evidence indicating that PET imaging with ^{68}Ga-somatostatin analogs and FDG PET may provide complementary information for evaluating pulmonary neuroendocrine tumors. It has been recommended that PET imaging with ^{68}Ga-somatostatin analogs should be the first choice and performed first in the initial evaluation of patients with clinical suspicion of pulmonary carcinoid, and, if negative, FDG PET/CT could be performed subsequently.[13] Large prospective studies analyses are needed to validate this diagnostic strategy.

PET IMAGING OF TUMOR PROLIFERATION

Uncontrolled cell proliferation is a key feature of malignancy. Increased cell division activity is an important prognosticator of various malignancies and an important target of anticancer treatment.

Ki-67 is a nuclear protein associated with cellular proliferation and is expressed in dividing phases of the cell cycle, namely the S, G1, G2, and M phases, but is not expressed in G0 phase. As a result, Ki-67 expression level is used as a marker for the proliferation of various tumors and is a critical feature that bears significant importance in cancer treatment. Lung cancers with high Ki-67 expression are associated with poor differentiation, decreased progression-free survival (PFS), and decreased overall survival (OS).[14–16] The Ki-67 proliferation index, defined as the percentage of cells with positive Ki-67 immunostaining in a section of confirmed carcinoma, is often used clinically but only from biopsy or surgically resected specimens.

FDG PET/CT has been used to correlate FDG activity with tumor proliferation. Multiple studies have suggested that the maximum standardized uptake value (SUVmax) of FDG PET/CT correlates with Ki-67 expression in patients with NSCLC.[16–19] Vesselle and colleagues[20] reported that Ki-67 expression (percentage of positive cells) correlates strongly with FDG uptake in NSCLC, especially in stage I lesions. Further investigation in a large, prospectively recruited cohort of 178 patients with potentially resectable NSCLC evaluated tumor histologic features and Ki-67 proliferation index. They found significant differences in NSCLC FDG uptake across histologic subtypes and differentiation groups, which paralleled nearly identical differences in Ki-67 scores, implying that FDG activity may indicate tumor cell proliferation status in NSCLC patients.[15] They also noted that tumor aggressiveness (as defined by Ki-67 expression level) is correlated with SUVmax but not with TNM stage.[15]

In contrast to FDG, 18F-fluorothymidine (FLT) is a PET tracer that directly targets cellular proliferation activity. FLT is a thymidine analog and is trapped in dividing cells during the S phase.[21] FLT is phosphorylated to 3-fluorothymidine monophosphate by thymidine kinase 1 and trapped intracellularly but not incorporated into DNA. Other thymidine analog, for example, 4'-[methyl-^{11}C]-thiothymidine ([11]C-4DST), has been developed as a cell proliferation PET marker based on the DNA incorporation rationale.[22]

FLT uptake in tumor cells correlates with Ki-67 expression, independent of cancer type or nature of sample.[23,24] FLT uptake in tumor cells also correlates with tumor angiogenesis[23] but not FDG activity.[25] FLT PET has a high specificity for detecting lung malignancies but with less accuracy for N staging in patients with lung cancer compared with FDG PET.[25,26]

FLT PET seems to have an important role in evaluating treatment response in patients with NSCLC.[27,28] Everitt and colleagues[28] prospectively evaluated cellular metabolism and proliferation in 20 patients with stages I to III NSCLC during radical chemoradiation therapy using serial FDG and FLT PET/CT (performed at baseline and during therapy [weeks 2 and 4]). They found that decrease in FLT activity is a more sensitive indicator of early treatment response than FDG activity changes.

FLT activity also has a prognostic value in NSCLC patients.[29,30] Kobe and colleagues[29] retrospectively evaluated the predictive value of early and late residual FDG and FLT uptake in 30 patients with stage IV NSCLC treated with erlotinib, with PET performed at 1 week (early) and 6 weeks (late) after the start of erlotinib treatment. Early and late residual FDG and FLT uptake were measured in up to 5 lesions per scan with different standardized uptake value (SUV) measurements and compared with short-term outcome (progression vs nonprogression after 6 weeks of erlotinib treatment). They found that nonprogression after 6 weeks was associated with significantly lower early and late residual FDG uptake but was not associated with early and late residual FLT uptake. In addition, early and late low residual FDG and FLT uptake in the course of erlotinib treatment was associated with improved PFS.

PET IMAGING OF HYPOXIA

Traditionally, the planning for clinical radiation treatment is based on the anatomic information regarding the localization and size of the tumor and the normal tissues around it, without taking into consideration tumor heterogeneity and other tumor microenvironment factors, such as hypoxia, which is associated with resistance to treatment and a poor outcome.

NSCLC tumors have significant interpatient and intratumor heterogeneity with regards to tissue hypoxia and metabolic activity.[31] Hypoxia is associated with resistance to radiotherapy and chemotherapy, requiring a 2.5-times to 3-times higher radiotherapy dose to achieve the same therapeutic effect for which accurate detection of the hypoxic region(s) within a tumor mass using PET imaging is helpful.[32] In addition, tumor hypoxia is a prognostic factor of treatment outcome in many types of cancer, including NSCLC. Noninvasive PET imaging of tumor hypoxia and heterogenous tumor oxygenation with a tumor mass is valuable to patient stratification and treatment adjustment.

There are multiple PET tracers to detect tissue hypoxia. 18F-fluoromisonidazole (FMISO) is the most studied hypoxia tracer. FMISO enters cells by passive diffusion. When the tissue oxygen level is low, FMISO is reduced, binds to intracellular macromolecules, and is trapped intracellularly.[33] In addition to SUV, tumor-to-blood uptake ratio and hypoxic fraction (the fraction of pixels within the imaged tumor volume) are used to quantify tumor hypoxia. FMISO, however, has slow accumulation in hypoxic tumors and slow background clearance with poor tumor-to-background contrast.

Incorporating hypoxia information from FMISO PET imaging into treatment planning could lead to improved treatment outcome while reducing irradiation side effects in surrounding normal tissues. It may also provide early identification of cases that might benefit from dose escalation or other counterhypoxic measures.[34] There is evidence that lower FMISO uptake is associated with better response to chemotherapy in patients with oral squamous cell carcinoma,[35] whereas higher accumulation of FMISO indicates an intratumoral hypoxic area.[36] Vera and colleagues[37] performed simultaneous PET imaging before and during radiotherapy in patients with biopsy-proved NSCLC to assess metabolism with FDG, proliferation with FLT, and hypoxia with FMISO. The 3 PET image sets were obtained in 5 patients before and during radiotherapy, with minimal intervals of 48 hours between each PET/CT scan. Both FLT SUVmax values and FDG SUVmax values were significantly lower ($P<.0006$) at scans during radiotherapy. A significant correlation was observed between FLT and FDG uptake ($r = 0.56$, $P<10[-4]$) and between FDG and FMISO uptakes ($r = 0.59$, $P = .0004$).

EGFR inhibition with erlotinib decreases expression of hypoxia-inducible factorv1-alpha and downstream expression of vascular endothelial growth factor (VEGF) and, as a result, reduces hypoxia in vivo. Arvold and colleagues[38] found that FMISO PET is able to detect changes in hypoxia in vivo in response to EGFR-targeted tyrosine kinase inhibitor (TKI) therapy in EGFR mutant NSCLC, both in mouse xenografts and in patients.

Another commonly used hypoxia PET tracer is Cu-diacetyl-bis(N4-methylthiosemicarbazone) (Cu-ATSM). Copper has several positron-emitting radioisotopes, including 64Cu (half-life [T1/2] 12.7 h), 62Cu (T1/2 9.7 min), and 60Cu (T1/2 24 min).[39] There is evidence that Cu-ATSM PET is promising in detecting tissue hypoxia in lung lesions[40] and may play a role as a prognostic marker in NSCLC patients.[41,42] Lopci and colleagues[42] performed a prospective recruitment of 18 consecutive patients with locally advanced NSCLC (n = 7) or head and neck cancer. These patients received Cu-ATSM PET, with a median follow-up period of 14.6 months. They observed that hypoxic tumor volume (HTV) ($P = .02$) and hypoxic burden (hypoxic burden = HTV × mean SUV) ($P = .05$) had a significant correlation to PFS. Other hypoxia PET tracers, such as 18F-fluoroazomycin arabinozide, also show prognostic value in NSCLC.[41,43] Although numerous PET tracers for hypoxia imaging have been investigated, most are still in early preclinical stages. As for those with clinical data, the sample sizes of those studies are often small, with limited pathologic and clinical correlations. In addition, the underlying mechanisms of radiotracer uptake and retention in hypoxic cells are not well understood for most hypoxia imaging tracers.[33] Further prospectively designed studies with larger sample sizes to correlate PET imaging findings with patient treatment strategies and outcomes are necessary.

PET IMAGING OF ANGIOGENESIS

Angiogenesis, or new blood vessel formation, is a physiologic process that may occur in numerous inflammatory conditions but is more prominent in malignancies. Angiogenesis associated with tumor growth is an interesting target for imaging diagnosis and for targeted therapy. Although other methods, such as dynamic contrast-enhanced CT and MR imaging, may be used for the assessment of tissue blood flow and perfusion that are related to angiogenesis, PET imaging has the advantage of targeting a molecular marker of angiogenic process and thus providing more specific assessments of angiogenic activity in tumors.

Radiolabeled integrin $\alpha v\beta 3$ antagonists have been the main interest in PET tracer development for imaging angiogenesis. Integrins (including $\alpha v\beta 3$) are a family of cell adhesion molecules up-regulated on activated endothelial cells and are involved in endothelial cell differentiation, growth, and migration. Integrin $\alpha v\beta 3$ binds to a variety of extracellular matrix molecules via the so-called arginine-glycine-aspartic acid (RGD) sequence with high affinity and specificity and plays an essential role in the regulation of tumor growth, regional invasiveness, and distant metastasis. The fact that the RGD peptide binds specifically with integrin $\alpha v\beta 3$ has attracted great interest, leading to development of a variety of radiolabeled RGD peptide tracers. Many studies have reported positive correlations of RGD-based tracer uptake with receptor density.[44,45] The assessment of $\alpha v\beta 3$ expression with 18F–galacto-RGD PET and of glucose metabolism with FDG PET in 18 patients with primary or metastatic cancer (including 10 NSCLC patients) revealed that there was no significant correlation between the SUVs for FDG and 18F–galacto-RGD either for all lesions, or for primary and metastatic lesions separately (P>.05). The lack of close correlation between tracer uptake of 18F–galacto-RGD and FDG in malignant lesions suggests a complementary role of RGD PET in addition to FDG PET evaluation in cancer patients.[46]

In addition to 18F, RGD peptides can be labeled with ^{68}Ga or ^{64}Cu for PET imaging. Zheng and colleagues[47] investigated the diagnostic value of a ^{68}Ga-labeled RGD PET tracer, ^{68}Ga–NOTA-PRGD2, for lung cancer; 91 patients with suspected lung lesions were enrolled and received ^{68}Ga–NOTA-PRGD2 PET/CT scan in addition to FDG PET/CT. ^{68}Ga–NOTA-PRGD2 was rapidly cleared from the blood pool. The SUVs of malignancies were significantly higher than those of benign lesions. The ^{68}Ga–NOTA-PRGD2 PET/CT had a similar diagnostic value for lung cancer compared with FDG PET/CT but demonstrated higher specificity than FDG PET/CT in assessing lymph node metastasis.

Preparation of 18F-labeled RGD peptides, however, suffers from multistep time-consuming steps and low yield. More recent developments of 18F-fluoride–aluminum complexes to label RDG peptides have led to the development of 18F–AlF-NOTA-PRGD2 (18F-alfatide).[48] It was shown that 18F-alfatide can be produced with excellent radiochemical yield and purity via a simple 1-step lyophilized kit with promising imaging properties and allows specific imaging of alphav-beta3 expression with good contrast in lung cancer patients.[49] Luan and colleagues[50] examined 18 patients with advanced NSCLC who had undergone 18F-alfatide PET/CT scans before concurrent chemoradiation therapy. They found that SUVmax, peak SUV, and tumor to normal tissue ratios were higher in nonresponders than in responders. Multivariate logistic regression analyses showed that tumor to normal lung uptake ratio was an independent predictor of the short-term outcome continuous renal replacement therapy in patients with advanced NSCLC (P = .032).

Another interesting PET imaging target for angiogenesis is VEGF. VEGF is a homodimeric glycoprotein with multiple isoforms. The binding of VEGF to VEGF tyrosine kinase receptors initiates a cascade of signaling pathways that mediate endothelial cell migration and proliferation.[51] Conventional therapy supplemented by VEGF inhibitors has demonstrated improvements in response, PFS, and/or OS in NSCLC and other malignancies.[52] Similarly, VEGF and VEGF receptors (VEGFRs) pathway has attracted significant

interest as a target for noninvasive PET imaging, which may be important in the early evaluation of antiangiogenic treatment efficacy of VEGFR-targeted therapy. Luo and colleagues[53] recently reported that 64Cu–NOTA-RamAb PET imaging revealed specific and prominent uptake of VEGFR-2–positive xenograft lung tumors and significantly lower uptake in VEGFR-2–negative tumors, suggesting promise for detecting VEGFR-2–positive malignancies and monitoring subsequent therapeutic response to VEGFR-2–targeted therapies.

Targeted molecular imaging of angiogenesis may offer critical information for NSCLC treatment. Most tracers in this area are at early stages of development and need considerable pharmacokinetic improvements. More importantly, clinical validation for these tracers is limited. More direct evidence is still needed that uptake of these tracers indicates tumor aggressiveness and that such uptake correlates with treatment response to guide treatment decisions.

PET TRACERS FOR TARGETED THERAPIES

Although clinical oncology has always been personalized, modern personalized medicine in clinical oncology has reached a new level in molecular genetics and signal pathway–specific targets, in addition to traditional consideration of patients' general health; cardiovascular, renal, and hepatic function; tumor subtypes and staging; and so forth. Research in driver oncogene mutations has seen rapid progress in recent years and has contributed to significant breakthroughs in therapeutic agents targeting some of these driver oncogenes. Traditionally, NSCLC is categorized by histologic subtypes, including adenocarcinoma, squamous cell carcinoma, and large cell carcinoma. Molecular diagnostics have now become part of routine clinical practice. In addition to histologic subtypes, the 2017 National Comprehensive Cancer Network (NCCN) Clinical Practice Guidelines in Oncology[54] recommend biomarker testing for EGFR mutation, ALK fusion oncogene/gene rearrangements, ROS1 gene rearrangements, and programmed death ligand-1 in patients with metastatic NSCLC.

The EGFR pathway is an important driver of tumor progression in various malignancies, including NSCLC, and great success has been reached using selective inhibitor of EGFR–tyrosine kinase domain as a therapeutic target.[55,56] The presence of activating EGFR mutations allows patient stratification for targeted drug treatment with TKIs (eg, erlotinib and gefitinib) in patients with advanced-stage NSCLC. Some EGFR mutations (such as exon 19 deletions and L858 R point mutation in exon 21, also called sensitizing mutations) are associated with significantly better response to EFGR–TKI therapy compared with conventional chemotherapy, whereas other mutations (such as exon 20 insertions) seem to be associated with resistance to EGFR inhibitors.[57] In addition, patients with KRAS mutations and ALK or ROS1 gene rearrangements are resistant to TKI therapy.

It is thus critically important to identify the presence of a molecular target before using molecularly targeted drugs to achieve optimal outcomes. Currently, genetic analysis of these driver genes and gene mutations is mainly conducted through in vitro DNA mutation detection assays, including direct DNA sequencing, polymerase chain reaction, and fluorescence in situ hybridization. Obtaining sufficient tumor tissue to perform these genetic analyses, however, is not always easy. Analysis from small biopsy specimens (often from a single tumor lesion) may miss tumor heterogeneity, especially for large tumor masses. More important, DNA sequencing and polymerase chain reaction, both based on a single sample of biopsy specimens, cannot provide in vivo information and do not provide 3-D distribution patterns.

The association between EGFR mutations in NSCLC and TKI therapy response highlights a potentially pivotal role that noninvasive molecular PET imaging may play in modern oncology. Previously, researchers have tried to link FDG PET findings to EGFR mutations. Findings thus far, however, have reached contradictory results. For example, Huang and colleagues[58] showed that patients with a high SUVmax were likely to have EGFR mutations. Meanwhile, other investigators have reported that high FDG avidity correlates with the EGFR wild-type genotype.[59,60] Chung and colleagues[61] found no significant differences in FDG PET/CT parameters (SUVmax, metabolic tumor volume, and total lesion glycolysis) between patients with or without EGFR mutation.

Still, novel PET tracers targeting the EGFR-TKI signaling pathway have achieved significant progress. Memon and colleagues[62] developed ^{11}C-erlotinib as a PET tracer that accumulates in EGFR-positive lung cancer xenografts in mice. In humans, ^{11}C-erlotinib PET/CT has been shown to detect NSCLC lung tumors, including lymph nodes not identified by FDG PET/CT, and is able to differentiate responders from nonresponders in NSCLC patients receiving erlotinib treatment.[63] Memon and colleagues[63] examined 13 patients with NSCLC destined for erlotinib treatment. These patients had ^{11}C-erlotinib PET/CT and FDG PET/CT prior to the start of erlotinib treatment

and underwent FDG PET/CT scans 12 weeks after erlotinib treatment. Patients with accumulations of ^{11}C-erlotinib had better outcomes after erlotinib therapy than those with no accumulation (3 of 4 patients with accumulation of ^{11}C-erlotinib showed a positive response to erlotinib treatment, whereas 7 of the 9 patients with no accumulation either died or had progressive disease and the other 2 had stable disease after 12 weeks of treatment).

[11]C-labeled 4-N-(3-bromoanilino)-6,7-dimethoxyquinazoline (^{11}C-PD153035) is another promising imaging biomarker of EGFR using PET. It specifically detects EGFR-TKI–sensitive cells/xenografts but not EGFR-TKI–resistant cells/xenografts.[64] ^{11}C-PD153035 has been shown to predict outcomes in patients with advanced chemotherapy-refractory NSCLC treated with EGFR-TKI and thus may be used for selection of patients likely to respond to the EGFR-TKI therapy. Meng and colleagues[65] evaluated 21 patients with advanced chemotherapy-refractory NSCLC, all prospectively enrolled on a trial of erlotinib and imaged by ^{11}C-PD153035 PET/CT at baseline, after 1 week to 2 weeks, and after 6 weeks of erlotinib treatment. They found that the baseline SUVmax correlated strongly with OS and PFS, independent of tumor histology. Patients with higher SUVmax (>median) survived more than twice as long (either OS or PFS) as patients with lower SUVmax. ^{11}C-PD153035 PET, however, was not good for monitoring treatment response, because uptake on follow-up scans was less well correlated with survival.

The ALK, an oncogenic receptor tyrosine kinase, belongs to a member of the insulin receptor superfamily. Various ALK fusion proteins resulting from chromosomal rearrangements have been implicated in the pathogenesis of several malignancies, including anaplastic large cell lymphoma, diffuse large B-cell lymphoma, and NSCLCs.[66] ALK has emerged as an important therapeutic target in solid and hematologic tumors. Multiple ALK inhibitors (crizotinib, ceritinib, and alectinib) are now Food and Drug Administration approved for the treatment of metastatic NSCLC in patients positive for ALK fusions.[67] On the other hand, drug resistance may occur (approximately 10 months after the initiation of therapy for crizotinib) when there are other unwanted mutations in the ALK fusion protein.[66] FDG PET/CT scans demonstrated that ALK-positive tumors had significantly higher FDG activity and were significantly less differentiated than ALK-negative tumors in patients with advanced lung adenocarcinoma.[68,69] Noninvasive direct imaging biomarkers of ALK fusion proteins, which are urgently needed for patient stratification, are not available. Perera and colleagues[70] recently synthesized a radiolabeled analog of the ALK inhibitor ceritinib, ^{18}F-fluoroethyl-ceritinib, as a PET tracer for the detection of ALK-overexpressing solid tumors, such as lung cancer. Further development in this field will significantly improve clinical practice of signal pathway targeted therapies.

SUMMARY

PET/CT is a unique imaging modality, allowing in vivo and quantitative analysis of functional status and at the molecular level. There has been increasing interest in developing new PET tracers beyond FDG with better sensitivity and specificity to improve lesion characterization, patient stratification, and therapeutic response monitoring. These new PET tracers target a unique aspect of tumor biology, such as cell proliferation, apoptosis, hypoxia, and angiogenesis, or a specific oncogene/signal pathway. The confirmation (and ideally, quantitative assessment) of some biomarkers for tumor heterogeneity and patient stratification may decide eventually if a therapy will succeed or fail. It is expected that in the near future, more PET imaging tracers targeting a specific aspect of tumor biology or signal pathway will be seen in clinical trials and eventually in routine clinical practice. This will establish an important cornerstone as the basis of personalized molecular therapy and change the practice of medicine in the future.

REFERENCES

1. Tamura M, Oda M, Matsumoto I, et al. Pattern and predictors of false positive lymph node involvement on positron emission tomography in patients with non-small cell lung cancer. Thorac Cardiovasc Surgeon 2012;60(2):105–10.
2. Li S, Zheng Q, Ma Y, et al. Implications of false negative and false positive diagnosis in lymph node staging of NSCLC by means of 18F-FDG PET/CT. PLoS One 2013;8(10):e78552.
3. Larsen JE, Minna JD. Molecular biology of lung cancer: clinical implications. Clin Chest Med 2011; 32(4):703–40.
4. Wolin EM. Advances in the diagnosis and management of well-differentiated and intermediate-differentiated neuroendocrine tumors of the lung. Chest 2017;151(5):1141–6.
5. Hendifar AE, Marchevsky AM, Tuli R. Neuroendocrine tumors of the lung: current challenges and advances in the diagnosis and management of well-differentiated disease. J Thorac Oncol 2017;12(3): 425–36.
6. Deppen SA, Blume J, Bobbey AJ, et al. 68Ga-DOTATATE Compared with 111In-DTPA-octreotide and conventional imaging for pulmonary and gastroenteropancreatic neuroendocrine tumors: a systematic review and meta-analysis. J Nucl Med 2016;57(6):872–8.
7. Venkitaraman B, Karunanithi S, Kumar A, et al. Role of 68Ga-DOTATOC PET/CT in initial evaluation of patients with suspected bronchopulmonary carcinoid. Eur J Nucl Med Mol Imaging 2014;41(5):856–64.
8. Walker R, Deppen S, Smith G, et al. 68Ga-DOTATATE PET/CT imaging of indeterminate pulmonary nodules and lung cancer. PLoS One 2017;12(2): e0171301.
9. Kuyumcu S, Adalet I, Sanli Y, et al. Somatostatin receptor scintigraphy with 111In-octreotide in pulmonary carcinoid tumours correlated with pathological and 18FDG PET/CT findings. Ann Nucl Med 2012; 26(9):689–97.
10. Kayani I, Conry BG, Groves AM, et al. A comparison of 68Ga-DOTATATE and 18F-FDG PET/CT in pulmonary neuroendocrine tumors. J Nucl Med 2009; 50(12):1927–32.
11. Kumar A, Jindal T, Dutta R, et al. Functional imaging in differentiating bronchial masses: an initial experience with a combination of (18)F-FDG PET-CT scan and (68)Ga DOTA-TOC PET-CT scan. Ann Nucl Med 2009;23(8):745–51.
12. Jindal T, Kumar A, Venkitaraman B, et al. Evaluation of the role of [18F]FDG-PET/CT and [68Ga] DOTATOC-PET/CT in differentiating typical and atypical pulmonary carcinoids. Cancer Imaging 2011;11:70–5.
13. Treglia G, Giovanella L, Lococo F. Evolving role of PET/CT with different tracers in the evaluation of pulmonary neuroendocrine tumours. Eur J Nucl Med Mol Imaging 2014;41(5):853–5.
14. Martin B, Paesmans M, Mascaux C, et al. Ki-67 expression and patients survival in lung cancer: systematic review of the literature with meta-analysis. Br J Cancer 2004;91(12):2018–25.
15. Vesselle H, Salskov A, Turcotte E, et al. Relationship between non-small cell lung cancer FDG uptake at PET, tumor histology, and Ki-67 proliferation index. J Thorac Oncol 2008;3(9):971–8.
16. Woo T, Okudela K, Yazawa T, et al. Prognostic value of KRAS mutations and Ki-67 expression in stage I lung adenocarcinomas. Lung Cancer 2009;65(3): 355–62.
17. Duhaylongsod FG, Lowe VJ, Patz EF Jr, et al. Lung tumor growth correlates with glucose metabolism measured by fluoride-18 fluorodeoxyglucose positron emission tomography. Ann Thorac Surg 1995; 60(5):1348–52.
18. Dooms C, van Baardwijk A, Verbeken E, et al. Association between 18F-fluoro-2-deoxy-D-glucose uptake values and tumor vitality: prognostic value of

positron emission tomography in early-stage non-small cell lung cancer. J Thorac Oncol 2009;4(7): 822–8.

19. Murakami S, Saito H, Sakuma Y, et al. Correlation of 18F-fluorodeoxyglucose uptake on positron emission tomography with Ki-67 index and pathological invasive area in lung adenocarcinomas 30 mm or less in size. Eur J Radiol 2010;75(2):e62–6.

20. Vesselle H, Schmidt RA, Pugsley JM, et al. Lung cancer proliferation correlates with [F-18] fluorodeoxyglucose uptake by positron emission tomography. Clin Cancer Res 2000;6(10):3837–44.

21. Buck AK, Halter G, Schirrmeister H, et al. Imaging proliferation in lung tumors with PET: 18F-FLT versus 18F-FDG. J Nucl Med 2003;44(9): 1426–31.

22. Minamimoto R, Toyohara J, Seike A, et al. 4'-[Methyl-11C]-thiothymidine PET/CT for proliferation imaging in non-small cell lung cancer. J Nucl Med 2012; 53(2):199–206.

23. Yang W, Zhang Y, Fu Z, et al. Imaging proliferation of 18F-FLT PET/CT correlated with the expression of microvessel density of tumour tissue in non-small-cell lung cancer. Eur J Nucl Med Mol Imaging 2012;39(8):1289–96.

24. Chalkidou A, Landau DB, Odell EW, et al. Correlation between Ki-67 immunohistochemistry and 18F-fluorothymidine uptake in patients with cancer: a systematic review and meta-analysis. Eur J Cancer 2012;48(18):3499–513.

25. Yang W, Zhang Y, Fu Z, et al. Imaging of proliferation with 18F-FLT PET/CT versus 18F-FDG PET/CT in non-small-cell lung cancer. Eur J Nucl Med Mol Imaging 2010;37(7):1291–9.

26. Buck AK, Hetzel M, Schirrmeister H, et al. Clinical relevance of imaging proliferative activity in lung nodules. Eur J Nucl Med Mol Imaging 2005;32(5): 525–33.

27. Trigonis I, Koh PK, Taylor B, et al. Early reduction in tumour [18F]fluorothymidine (FLT) uptake in patients with non-small cell lung cancer (NSCLC) treated with radiotherapy alone. Eur J Nucl Med Mol Imaging 2014;41(4):682–93.

28. Everitt SJ, Ball DL, Hicks RJ, et al. Differential (18) F-FDG and (18)F-FLT uptake on serial PET/CT imaging before and during definitive chemoradiation for non-small cell lung cancer. J Nucl Med 2014;55(7): 1069–74.

29. Kobe C, Scheffler M, Holstein A, et al. Predictive value of early and late residual 18F-fluorodeoxyglucose and 18F-fluorothymidine uptake using different SUV measurements in patients with non-small-cell lung cancer treated with erlotinib. Eur J Nucl Med Mol Imaging 2012;39(7):1117–27.

30. Scheffler M, Zander T, Nogova L, et al. Prognostic impact of [18F]fluorothymidine and [18F]fluoro-D-glucose baseline uptakes in patients with lung cancer treated first-line with erlotinib. PLoS One 2013;8(1):e53081.

31. van Elmpt W, Zegers CML, Reymen B, et al. Multiparametric imaging of patient and tumour heterogeneity in non-small-cell lung cancer: quantification of tumour hypoxia, metabolism and perfusion. Eur J Nucl Med Mol Imaging 2016;43(2):240–8.

32. Szyszko TA, Yip C, Szlosarek P, et al. The role of new PET tracers for lung cancer. Lung Cancer 2016;94: 7–14.

33. Yip C, Blower PJ, Goh V, et al. Molecular imaging of hypoxia in non-small-cell lung cancer. Eur J Nucl Med Mol Imaging 2015;42(6):956–76.

34. Toma-Dasu I, Uhrdin J, Antonovic L, et al. Dose prescription and treatment planning based on FMISO-PET hypoxia. Acta Oncologica 2012;51(2): 222–30.

35. Sato J, Kitagawa Y, Yamazaki Y, et al. Advantage of FMISO-PET over FDG-PET for predicting histological response to preoperative chemotherapy in patients with oral squamous cell carcinoma. Eur J Nucl Med Mol Imaging 2014;41(11):2031–41.

36. Tachibana I, Nishimura Y, Shibata T, et al. A prospective clinical trial of tumor hypoxia imaging with 18F-fluoromisonidazole positron emission tomography and computed tomography (F-MISO PET/CT) before and during radiation therapy. J Radiat Res 2013;54(6):1078–84.

37. Vera P, Bohn P, Edet-Sanson A, et al. Simultaneous positron emission tomography (PET) assessment of metabolism with 18F-fluoro-2-deoxy-d-glucose (FDG), proliferation with 18F-fluoro-thymidine (FLT), and hypoxia with 18fluoro-misonidazole (F-miso) before and during radiotherapy in patients with non-small-cell lung cancer (NSCLC): a pilot study. Radiother Oncol 2011;98(1):109–16.

38. Arvold ND, Heidari P, Kunawudhi A, et al. Tumor hypoxia response after targeted therapy in EGFR-mutant non-small cell lung cancer: proof of concept for FMISO-PET. Technol Cancer Res Treat 2016; 15(2):234–42.

39. Laforest R, Dehdashti F, Lewis JS, et al. Dosimetry of 60/61/62/64Cu-ATSM: a hypoxia imaging agent for PET. Eur J Nucl Med Mol Imaging 2005;32(7): 764–70.

40. Zhang T, Das SK, Fels DR, et al. PET with 62Cu-ATSM and 62Cu-PTSM is a useful imaging tool for hypoxia and perfusion in pulmonary lesions. AJR Am J Roentgenology 2013;201(5):W698–706.

41. Kinoshita T, Fujii H, Hayashi Y, et al. Prognostic significance of hypoxic PET using (18)F-FAZA and (62) Cu-ATSM in non-small-cell lung cancer. Lung Cancer 2016;91:56–66.

42. Lopci E, Grassi I, Rubello D, et al. Prognostic evaluation of disease outcome in solid tumors investigated with 64Cu-ATSM PET/CT. Clin Nucl Med 2016;41(2):e87–92.

43. Saga T, Inubushi M, Koizumi M, et al. Prognostic value of (18) F-fluoroazomycin arabinoside PET/CT in patients with advanced non-small-cell lung cancer. Cancer Sci 2015;106(11):1554–60.

44. Chen X, Sievers E, Hou Y, et al. Integrin alpha v beta 3-targeted imaging of lung cancer. Neoplasia 2005; 7(3):271–9.

45. Haubner R. Alphavbeta3-integrin imaging: a new approach to characterise angiogenesis? Eur J Nucl Med Mol Imaging 2006;33(Suppl 1):54–63.

46. Beer AJ, Lorenzen S, Metz S, et al. Comparison of integrin alphaVbeta3 expression and glucose metabolism in primary and metastatic lesions in cancer patients: a PET study using 18F-galacto-RGD and 18F-FDG. J Nucl Med 2008;49(1):22–9.

47. Zheng K, Liang N, Zhang J, et al. 68Ga-NOTA-PRGD2 PET/CT for integrin imaging in patients with lung cancer. J Nucl Med 2015;56(12):1823–7.

48. Lang L, Li W, Guo N, et al. Comparison study of [18F] FAl-NOTA-PRGD2, [18F]FPPRGD2, and [68Ga]Ga-NOTA-PRGD2 for PET imaging of U87MG tumors in mice. Bioconjug Chem 2011;22(12):2415–22.

49. Wan W, Guo N, Pan D, et al. First experience of 18F-alfatide in lung cancer patients using a new lyophilized kit for rapid radiofluorination. J Nucl Med 2013;54(5):691–8.

50. Luan X, Huang Y, Gao S, et al. 18F-alfatide PET/CT may predict short-term outcome of concurrent chemoradiotherapy in patients with advanced non-small cell lung cancer. Eur J Nucl Med Mol Imaging 2016;43(13):2336–42.

51. Murukesh N, Dive C, Jayson GC. Biomarkers of angiogenesis and their role in the development of VEGF inhibitors. Br J Cancer 2010;102(1):8–18.

52. Liang W, Wu X, Hong S, et al. Multi-targeted antiangiogenic tyrosine kinase inhibitors in advanced non-small cell lung cancer: meta-analyses of 20 randomized controlled trials and subgroup analyses. PLoS One 2014;9(10):e109757.

53. Luo H, England CG, Graves SA, et al. PET Imaging of VEGFR-2 expression in lung cancer with 64Cu-labeled ramucirumab. J Nucl Med 2016;57(2):285–90.

54. Ettinger DS, Wood DE, Aisner DL, et al. Non-small cell lung cancer, version 5.2017, NCCN clinical practice guidelines in oncology. J Natl Compr Canc Netw 2017;15(4):504–35.

55. Su Z. Epidermal growth factor receptor mutation-guided treatment for lung cancers: where are we now? Thorac Cancer 2011;2(1):1–6.

56. Liao BC, Lin CC, Yang JC. Novel EGFR Inhibitors in non-small cell lung cancer: current status of afatinib. Curr Oncol Rep 2017;19(1):4.

57. Gazdar AF. Activating and resistance mutations of EGFR in non-small-cell lung cancer: role in clinical response to EGFR tyrosine kinase inhibitors. Oncogene 2009;28(Suppl 1):S24–31.

58. Huang CT, Yen RF, Cheng MF, et al. Correlation of F-18 fluorodeoxyglucose-positron emission tomography maximal standardized uptake value and EGFR mutations in advanced lung adenocarcinoma. Med Oncol 2010;27(1):9–15.

59. Mak RH, Digumarthy SR, Muzikansky A, et al. Role of 18F-fluorodeoxyglucose positron emission tomography in predicting epidermal growth factor receptor mutations in non-small cell lung cancer. Oncologist 2011;16(3):319–26.

60. Putora PM, Fruh M, Muller J. FDG-PET SUV-max values do not correlate with epidermal growth factor receptor mutation status in lung adenocarcinoma. Respirology 2013;18(4):734–5.

61. Chung HW, Lee KY, Kim HJ, et al. FDG PET/CT metabolic tumor volume and total lesion glycolysis predict prognosis in patients with advanced lung adenocarcinoma. J Cancer Res Clin Oncol 2014; 140(1):89–98.

62. Memon AA, Jakobsen S, Dagnaes-Hansen F, et al. Positron emission tomography (PET) imaging with [11C]-labeled erlotinib: a micro-PET study on mice with lung tumor xenografts. Cancer Res 2009; 69(3):873–8.

63. Memon AA, Weber B, Winterdahl M, et al. PET imaging of patients with non-small cell lung cancer employing an EGF receptor targeting drug as tracer. Br J Cancer 2011;105(12):1850–5.

64. Dai D, Li X-F, Wang J, et al. Predictive efficacy of (11)C-PD153035 PET imaging for EGFR-tyrosine kinase inhibitor sensitivity in non-small cell lung cancer patients. Int J Cancer 2016;138(4):1003–12.

65. Meng X, Loo BW Jr, Ma L, et al. Molecular imaging with 11C-PD153035 PET/CT predicts survival in non-small cell lung cancer treated with EGFR-TKI: a pilot study. J Nucl Med 2011;52(10): 1573–9.

66. Roskoski R Jr. Anaplastic lymphoma kinase (ALK): structure, oncogenic activation, and pharmacological inhibition. Pharmacol Res 2013;68(1):68–94.

67. Holla VR, Elamin YY, Bailey AM, et al. ALK: a tyrosine kinase target for cancer therapy. Cold Spring Harb Mol Case Stud 2017;3(1):a001115.

68. Choi H, Paeng JC, Kim D-W, et al. Metabolic and metastatic characteristics of ALK-rearranged lung adenocarcinoma on FDG PET/CT. Lung Cancer 2013;79(3):242–7.

69. Jeong CJ, Lee HY, Han J, et al. Role of imaging biomarkers in predicting anaplastic lymphoma kinase-positive lung adenocarcinoma. Clin Nucl Med 2015;40(1):e34–9.

70. Perera S, Piwnica-Worms D, Alauddin MM. Synthesis of a [(18)F]-labeled ceritinib analogue for positron emission tomography of anaplastic lymphoma kinase, a receptor tyrosine kinase, in lung cancer. J Labelled Comp Radiopharm 2016;59(3):103–8.

Future Directions in PET Imaging of Lung Cancer

Tim Akhurst, MBBS, FRACP

KEYWORDS

- Non–small cell lung cancer • Food and Drug Administration • Response assessment
- Radiochemistry

KEY POINTS

- Malignancy and the inflammatory response both are energy dependant, and FDG avid. This makes FDG nonspecific.
- Population based statistics tell us nothing about how an individual patient will respond to a particular therapy, molecular imaging should fill this gap as it interrogates the whole patient, but specific biomarkers are needed.
- Thousands of PET tracers have been developed, most languish on laboratory shelves, this lack of translation to clinical use is an indictment of the efficacy of the approval processes worldwide.
- Many new cancer therapeutics are extremely expensive, this changes the economics of medical imaging, and offers the opportunity for incorporation of imaging into the rational use of these agents.

INTRODUCTION

The unmet needs of PET imaging of lung cancer are (1) differentiating inflammatory change from tumor; (2) prediction of a lack of response to cell-cycle–specific therapy, such as radiation and chemotherapy before treatment commences; (3) prediction of response to expensive therapies, such as programmed cell death protein 1 (PD-1) inhibition; (4) more uniform reimbursement for novel imaging agents; (5) new theranostic paradigms; (6) hardware advances; and (7) integration of PET into phase III drug trials.

INFLAMMATION OR TUMOR?

An ongoing issue regarding ^{18}F 2-fluoro-2-deoxy-D-glucose (FDG) imaging of lung cancer is the lack of specificity of FDG. Any physiologic response to a local insult is typically associated with increased use of glucose to provide the fuel to power the response. Larson[1] wrote an editorial regarding this topic in 1994; it seems that more than 20 years later solving this problem is still some ways away.

Inflammatory changes can be drug related; in particular, newer methods of treating cancer involving immunomodulation can have associated autoimmune effects that are detectable with FDG.[2] Inflammatory changes can be related to radiation. It is known that radiation of normal lung causes radiation pneumonitis; early phases of this response to therapy are typically quite FDG avid. In the past, radiotherapy of lung cancer typically involved posteroanterior/anteroposterior fields with or without lateral fields; the fields, therefore, had sharp cutoffs whose linear nature did not correspond to expected anatomic structures. As radiation therapy become more conformal, the radiation-induced inflammatory changes seen are

---

Disclosures: None.

Nuclear Medicine Service, Cancer Imaging, Peter MacCallum Cancer Centre, University of Melbourne, 305 Grattan Street, Melbourne, Victoria 3000, Australia

E-mail address: tim.akhurst@petermac.org

PET Clin 13 (2018) 83–88

https://doi.org/10.1016/j.cpet.2017.09.005

also becoming more lump-like rather than regional, making morphology of change less reliable in assigning FDG activity as a reactive process; with the passage of time, the predictive accuracy of focal FDG uptake increases.[3]

Image registration based on 2 CT data sets is becoming routine, and, using the CT data as a template, disparate emission data sets can be registered. If a specific radiopharmaceutical could be developed that would image host inflammatory processes, a subtraction technique could highlight areas concerning for malignancy.

Some infectious agents themselves are exquisitely FDG avid; as an example, *Cryptococcus neoformans* itself typically has high FDG uptake, and this may underlie its pathogenesis.[4] Dual-tracer techniques that are specific for particular infectious agents is another approach that could be used now; for example, [68]gallium citrate could be used to image pneumocystis.[5]

There is a clear unmet need for agents that specifically image inflammation that would allow more specific interpretation of FDG uptake and improve patient care, particularly with regard to the mediastinal nodes.

PRETREATMENT RESPONSE PREDICTION

Treatments fail if the therapy is the wrong target or if it is delivered to the wrong place or in an incorrect amount. Some of the resistance to therapy is, therefore, mechanical, with poor penetration or high efflux, or biological, with cells essentially ignoring a message to die. The mechanistic questions can be answered with a tracer technique, and PET imaging is ideally suited to this task. The biological questions requires a surrogate biomarker to be developed.

Moehler and colleagues[6] reported the utility of F-18–labeled fluorouracil PET, and the uptake and retention of the tracer at 120 minutes was predictive of response to 5-fluorouracil chemotherapy for colon cancer liver metastases. Importantly they found intrapatient, interlesional heterogeneity of uptake. This heterogeneity underpins the rationale for an imaging technique rather than a reliance on genomics because single samples will never reflect the status of all tumor within a patient. Chiosis chose to design and develop an heat shock protein 90 (HSP-90) inhibitor that contained an iodine atom such that a chemically identical compound radiolabeled with [124]Iodine was codeveloped to allow in vivo pharmacokinetics of the therapeutics to be assessed as the drug passed through the various phases of clinical testing.[7] Although cisplatin has been radiolabeled, there are no articles describing such compounds in the clinic. A literature search found no articles describing radiolabeled gemcitabine. Therefore, the field of imaging the pharmacokinetics of commonly used cytotoxic chemotherapy used in lung cancer is as yet unexplored.

Prior efforts to image incipient cell death using annexin have not translated into clinical oncology, probably because of the utility of FDG to image viable cells, and the absence of a response on FDG is likely equally as important a signal showing cell death is occurring. Several PET imaging agents have been synthesized that are variants of annexin. Immunomodulatory agents have recently revolutionized the treatment of melanoma, with dramatic responses seen with durable responses seen in some patients. Such agents are not as successful in lung cancer; nevertheless, prolonged and durable responses are seen in some patients. These agents are expensive, costing tens of thousands of dollars per dose. In designing an agent that predicts response to PD-1 or programmed death-ligand-1 (PDL-1) agents, it is important to remember that there are multiple aspects of tumor and host that need to be present for the agents to be needed and successful. As an example, if the required T cells are not present or do not express PD-1, no amount of unmasking of the tumor with drug leads to a response. Similarly, if the tumor does not express PDL-1, then a PD-1 inhibitor can have no effect. There are preclinical agents imaging PD-1[8] on lymphocytes and PDL-1[9] on tumors.

INTEGRATION OF FUNCTIONAL IMAGING INTO CLINICAL TRIALS

The number of ground-breaking clinical trials describing improvements in patient outcomes related to new drugs that have integrated functional imaging within the trial is dreadfully low. There are several reasons behind this. A pharmaceutical company is a business whose primary role is to make money for its shareholders. The products sold are a route to this goal. It is not in the company's interests to develop biomarkers that limit the number of patients who are administered their products. The governmental mandate for drug development and approval is safety and efficacy with no concern for cost, and as long as some patients benefit, drugs are often approved. Drug companies design clinical trials to comply with these demands. Drug company executives do not perform science for science's sake and to limit costs, biomarker imaging endpoints are often excluded from trial design. Unless imaging biomarkers are made a requirement for approval and funding, drug companies are actually not acting in shareholder's interests in including them in trial design. PET imaging endpoints are not universally embraced/agreed on and the plethora of endpoints weakness the case for PET imaging to be included in clinical trials.

There is some community resistance to ever-increasing drug costs, with a seminal op-ed published in the *New York Times* justifying the Memorial Sloan Kettering Cancer Center decision to not to introduce a new drug into the hospital's formulary based on its cost and lack of improvement over existing therapies.[10] Nobody is suggesting that patients should be denied access to drugs that are effective, but when only 20% of patients have a durable response, the actual cost of the drug per effective treatment is actually 5 times higher than the published cost per patient. The high cost of new drugs is making the invention of accurate biomarkers more attractive; a diagnostic test costing thousands of dollars can make economic sense if it limits the use of a drug costing tens of thousands of dollars. As discussed previously, tumor heterogeneity can limit the value of histopathologic or genomic biomarkers; this is something that PET can overcome because PET is the most sensitive whole-biomarker technique. The nuclear medicine community must convince their oncology colleagues and regulatory bodies to mandate the incorporation of PET imaging into phase III clinical trials so that drugs can be prescribed to enriched populations where the probability of response is highest.

ALTERNATIVE APPROVAL AND FUNDING FOR NOVEL PET AGENTS

The explosion of understanding of tumor biology has led to a massive increase in the number of targets that are exploitable and potentially imageable. Ten years ago, the US Department of Energy and the National Institutes of Health asked the National Academy of Sciences, the National Academy of Engineering, and the Institute of Medicine to review the state of the science of nuclear medicine. Their report[11] suggested changes needed to be made to simplify the approval process for diagnostic imaging agents; 10 years on, significant barriers remain. To understand the relative risks to the community of a new radiopharmaceutical, it is important to understand the population at risk; in 2009, there were 567,628 deaths from cancer in the United States.[12] Taken across the 10 years since the National Academies' report, approximately 6 million cancer deaths have occurred. Of the 1625 PET agents in the Molecular Imaging and Contrast Agent Database (https://www.ncbi.nlm.nih.gov/books/NBK5330) at the time of its final update (June 27, 2013), fewer than a dozen agents have current Food and Drug Administration

approval. There is a clear breakdown in translation of the inventiveness of basic science researchers into clinical practice. The National Oncology PET Registry study documented approximately 30% positive impact of FDG imaging across all types of cancer.[13] From a societal perspective, there would have to be a dramatic incidence of death related to a new radiopharmaceutical to make the net effect of unfettered access to novel radiopharmaceuticals a negative. The biggest barriers to routine translation of preclinical imaging research into the clinic are the financial and legalistic strangulation of ideas, based on a lack of funding and the hurdles placed in front of attempts to license new imaging technologies. If advancing the field is truly desired, these barriers need to be broken down. There are costs involved in performing a PET scan; they can be categorized into fixed costs of plant and equipment, per-scan costs of consumables, and labor. If a divorce from a single rebate for a single procedure can be achieved, then modular funding models could be created that would reimburse for a PET scan, taking into consideration the radiopharmaceutical cost. Microfluidics offers a potential new method of licensing, whereby a kit is licensed; and, within mandated activities of radioisotope and classes and amounts (in micrograms or less) of molecules, rapid approvals could be given for new radiopeptides. As an example, somatostatin analogs as a class can be coupled with a variety of approved chelators with a variety of radiometals. Approval for in human use for variations in the parent molecule could be based on in vitro stability. This means that ^{64}copper-labeled radiopharmaceuticals could be substituted for ^{111}indium and ^{68}gallium-labeled radiopharmaceuticals, and the payment for the imaging could be based on the agreed price of the kit and the fixed facility fee for the imaging. If a new peptide, for example, targeting prostate-specific membrane antigen, was shown to have acceptable stability when radiolabeled with a kit in vitro, it should be automatically approved for human use in pilot studies whose endpoint would be exclusion of alterations in physiologic parameters, such as variations in blood pressure, pulse rate, and oxygenation. These studies could use a nonradioactive form of the radiopharmaceutical. The argument for licensing of this type is that the microgram doses of peptide are unlikely to have any pharmacologic effect, and the kit form of radiolabeling is more reliable than bench based radiolabeling because it is less operator dependent. This template of funding and licensing would allow a rapid rollout of new radiopharmaceuticals, and then trials and or market forces can determine if the compound is clinically useful.

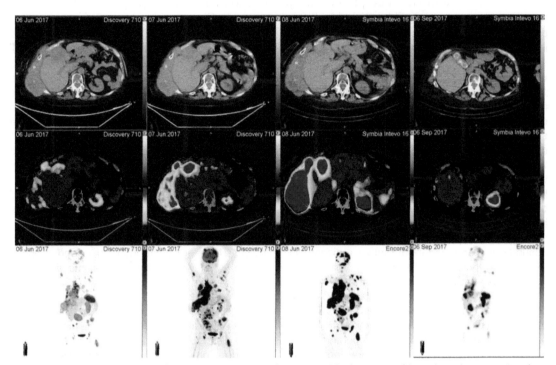

Fig. 1. This 68 year old non smoking woman presented in 2013 with shortness of breath and an anterior chest wall mass and initial investigations revealed a poorly differentiated malignancy, diffusely staining with squamous cell markers CD5/6 suggestive of a lung cancer. She had chest wall involvement at diagnosis and was offered palliative radiotherapy. It was noted during radiation therapy that the tumor responded rapidly. She consented to chemotherapy with gemcitabine and carboplatin. Follow up imaging revealed chest wall progression and this too was irradiated, with prompt local control. She was then placed on Nivolumab as her tumour expressed PDL-1. In May of 2017, she developed somnolence and an MRI revealed exophytic dural metastases. These lesions were debulked but were unresectable due to disease extent. Histopathology on the resected specimen revealed neuroendocrine features, with diffuse staining with synaptophysin, a new finding compared to 2013. A [68]Gallium-dota-Octreotate scan was performed this revealed acceptable uptake and so an FDG scan was performed to exclude discordant disease. The patient was offered whole brain radiation but chose PRRT, as other sites of disease were also progressing. She has received 3 cycles of [177]Lutetium-dota-Octreotate. The images are arranged vertically from each acquisition. The left panels are the initial [68]Gallium-dota-Octreotate images, showing a large chest wall lesion with extensive metastases, seen in the MIP images in the lowest row. The baseline ^{18}F-FDG scan is in the second panel from the left. The third panel is the 18 hour post [177]Lutetium-dota-Octreotate images. Notice how there is good correlation of the Gallium and Lutetium images. The images in the right most panels are also 18 hour post [177]Lutetium-dota-Octreotate images this time from the third PRRTT administration and show the effects of the first two cycles of therapy. Notice the reduction in the size of the lesion in the right chest wall. The increased intensity of the post treatment uptake is due to debulking of the FDG avid components of the disease, with residual lower grade tumor remaining. The patient has had no side effects related to her PRRT. The patient has also been spared the time and toxicity associated with whole brain irradiation.

NEW INSTRUMENTATION

PET CT is established, PET MR imaging is becoming so, and there are some exciting devices being developed, with whole-body (2-m) fields of view. These devices allow whole-body imaging within minutes if desired or dramatic reductions in administered dose. The other potential of these whole-body devices is the rapid assessment of new radiopharmaceuticals with whole-body pharmacokinetic studies easily acquired. There have been advances in the CT space as well, with dual-energy CT devices deployed worldwide. In terms of PET, a dual-energy CT device, by accurately mapping mu values rather than Hounsfield units, should enable more scaling of the CT data into the 511-keV energy that is required for true attenuation correct as was previously attainable with [68]Germanium/[68]Gallium rod sources. This should bring PET back to the truly quantitative device it previously was.[14,15]

THERANOSTICS

Many patients prescribed targeted agents, such as tyrosine kinase inhibitors, relapse with new mutations that confer resistance. This is biodiversity at work with outgrowth of cells that are not inhibited by the drug. Some approaches to overcome this involve conjugating the drug with another more toxic drug. A recent article from the Memorial Sloan Kettering Cancer Center is seminal in that it demonstrates the use of radioactive iodine augmenting the use of a MEK inhibitor.[16] The most important concept of the article is the demonstration of the combination of the recognition of a genetic abnormality for which a targeted agent is available and the use of a cytotoxic agent that acts beyond the cell in which it resides. The use of radioactivity is likely to be more effective than other options, such as drug conjugates, because the drug, once released from its vehicle, can rapidly elute whereas radioactive elements residing in a cell can continue to irradiate the local area.

The concept that a therapeutic, diagnostic (theranostic) pair can be developed and brought to the clinic has been shown to be incredibly powerful. The best known theranostic paradigm is based on the somatostatin receptor (SSR). The treatment is called peptide receptor radionuclide therapy (PRRT). The concept is that the SSR diagnostic agent, be it [111]indium or [68]gallium, predicts where the therapeutic radiopharmaceutical will deliver its energy. There is increasing recognition that FDG PET has a role in determining the likely efficacy of PRRT. FDG has 2 roles. The first is predicting the aggressiveness of the tumor, with the amount of FDG uptake predicting the degree of differentiation of the tumor. In general, neuroendocrine tumors without FDG uptake progress more slowly than those with FDG uptake, giving some understanding of the urgency of the need to treat. The second role is in determining the presence or absence of deposits of tumor that are remote from the deposits that are SSR positive, a phenomenon labeled spatial discordance. The presence of spatially discordant disease leaves those deposits hidden from the radiation delivered and, therefore, free to grow unfettered; unless a discordant lesion can be otherwise ablated, patients with discordant disease are unsuitable for PRRT. Thoracic malignancies variably express SSRs; when they are present, responses can be seen similar to other neuroendocrine tumors arising in other organs. When present, responses to PRRT can be dramatic (**Fig. 1**). Lung cancers are vulnerable to radiation. A future direction for PET in lung cancer should be in developing new theranostic paradigms based on driver mutations to not just suppress but kill cells and their neighbors based on targetable proteins specific to the mutation in question.

SUMMARY

There is an ongoing and successful effort in developing new radiopharmaceuticals that coupled with new developments in chemistry and instrumentation offers the potential of rapidly defining imaging biomarkers and theranostic paradigms. The overarching challenge remains in funding and approving such agents; the Food and Drug Administration in the United States is making efforts to improve the process, but the time to release PET agents from the regulator shackles is surely now, to bring to patients the excellence of preclinical work that has already been done.

REFERENCES

1. Larson SM. Cancer or inflammation? A Holy Grail for nuclear medicine. J Nucl Med 1994;35(10):1653–5.
2. Goethals L, Wilgenhof S, De Geeter F, et al. 18F-FDG PET/CT imaging of an anti-CTLA-4 antibody-associated autoimmune pancolitis. Eur J Nucl Med Mol Imaging 2011;38(7):1390–1.
3. Nakajima N, Sugawara Y, Kataoka M, et al. Differentiation of tumor recurrence from radiation-induced pulmonary fibrosis after stereotactic ablative radiotherapy for lung cancer: characterization of 18F-FDG PET/CT findings. Ann Nucl Med 2013;27(3): 261–70.
4. Price MS, Betancourt-Quiroz M, Price JL, et al. Cryptococcus neoformans requires a functional glycolytic pathway for disease but not persistence in the host. MBio 2011;2(3):e00103–11.
5. Levenson SM, Warren RD, Richman SD, et al. Abnormal pulmonary gallium accumulation in P. carinii pneumonia. Radiology 1976;119(2):395–8.
6. Moehler M, Dimitrakopoulou-Strauss A, Gutzler F, et al. 18F-labeled fluorouracil positron emission tomography and the prognoses of colorectal carcinoma patients with metastases to the liver treated with 5-fluorouracil. Cancer 1998;83(2):245–53.
7. Taldone T, Zatorska D, Ochiana SO, et al. Radiosynthesis of the iodine-124 labeled Hsp90.inhibitor PU-H71. J Labelled Comp Radiopharm 2016;59(3): 129–32.
8. Natarajan A, Mayer AT, Xu L, et al. Novel radiotracer for ImmunoPET imaging of PD-1 checkpoint expression on tumor infiltrating lymphocytes. Bioconjug Chem 2015;26(10):2062–9.
9. Heskamp S, Hobo W, Molkenboer-Kuenen JD, et al. Noninvasive imaging of tumor PD-L1 expression using radiolabeled anti-PD-L1 antibodies. Cancer Res 2015;75(14):2928–36.
10. Bach PB, Saltz LB, Wittes RE. In cancer care, cost matters. New York Times 2012.
11. National Research C, Institute of Medicine Committee on State of the Science of Nuclear M. The National

Academies collection: reports funded by National Institutes of Health. In: Advancing nuclear medicine through innovation. Washington, DC: National Academies Press (US) National Academy of Sciences; 2007. Available at: https://www.nap.edu/catalog/11985/advancing-nuclear-medicine-through-innovation.

12. Siegel R, Naishadham D, Jemal A. Cancer statistics, 2013. CA Cancer J Clin 2013;63(1):11–30.

13. Hillner BE, Siegel BA, Liu D, et al. Impact of positron emission tomography/computed tomography and positron emission tomography (PET) alone on expected management of patients with cancer: initial results from the National Oncologic PET Registry. J Clin Oncol 2008;26(13):2155–61.

14. Patrick JC, Terry Thompson R, So A, et al. Technical note: comparison of megavoltage, dual-energy, and single-energy CT-based mu-maps for a four-channel breast coil in PET/MRI. Med Phys 2017; 44(9):4758–65.

15. Rehfeld NS, Heismann BJ, Kupferschlager J, et al. Single and dual energy attenuation correction in PET/CT in the presence of iodine based contrast agents. Med Phys 2008;35(5):1959–69.

16. Ho AL, Grewal RK, Leboeuf R, et al. Selumetinib-enhanced radioiodine uptake in advanced thyroid cancer. N Engl J Med 2013;368(7):623–32.

Improved Detection of Small Pulmonary Nodules Through Simultaneous MR/PET Imaging

CrossMark

Fernando E. Boada, PhD*, Thomas Koesters, PhD,
Kai Tobias Block, PhD, Hersh Chandarana, MD

KEYWORDS

- MR/PET • Lung nodule • Motion correction

KEY POINTS

- Assessment of small lung nodules is challenging because of the significant blur due to respiratory (and often nonperiodic motion).
- Tracking respiratory motion during PET/computed tomography and MR/PET imaging using external devices is limited because of the small dynamic range of the devices and the inherent assumption that the respiratory motion is periodic throughout the examination.
- Prospective respiratory motion tracking and correction does not require the motion to be periodic and, as a result, leads to improved quantitative assessment of standard uptake values for small pulmonary nodules.

INTRODUCTION

The development of the MR/PET imaging platform provides, for the first time, a true synergistic imaging platform whereby information from each of the component modalities can be used to improve their individual image quality. Examples would be the use of high-resolution MR imaging scans to improve the quality of the PET images[1] or the use of PET images to reject undersampling artifacts from highly undersampled dynamic MR imaging scans.[2] The installed base of MR/PET systems is currently relatively small. However, the complementary nature of the information provided by the two modalities together with the synergisms implicit in collecting simultaneous information have allowed this platform to become the preferred choice for the diagnosis of conditions, such as dementia, neurofibromatosis, and epilepsy. For oncologic imaging, there are several applications whereby the MR/PET technology is poised to make significant improvements because of its improved workflow and capabilities. One of the oncologic applications that might benefit greatly from the capabilities of a simultaneous MR/PET acquisition is lung cancer. Lung cancer is the leading cause of cancer-related death in the Western world. Early detection of lung cancer is challenging, as the symptoms are often very similar to those of other common respiratory ailments. Multidetector computed tomography (MDCT) is routinely used for evaluation of disease in the lung and can be routinely performed without intravenous contrast administration and with a low radiation dose.[3] Although MDCT has

This article originally appeared in *Magnetic Resonance Imaging Clinics*, Volume 25, Issue 2, May 2017.
Disclosure Statement: The authors have nothing to disclose.
Department of Radiology, Center for Advanced Imaging Innovation and Research, New York University Langone Medical Center, 660 First Avenue, New York, NY 10016, USA
* Corresponding author.
E-mail address: Fernando.Boada@nyumc.org

high sensitivity for nodule detection, it has limited specificity in discriminating malignant from benign nodules even in setting of primary malignancy.[4] Assessment of metabolic activity within lung nodules with fludeoxyglucose F18 (18F-FDG) PET is often improved when compared with computed tomography (CT) for discriminating benign from malignant nodules,[5,6] making PET/CT the preferred modality to assess whole-body metastatic burden in many primary malignancies.

However, there are concerns with respect to the accuracy of PET/CT in the detection and characterization of subcentimeter pulmonary. Specifically, nodules of less than 1 cm in diameter have a high (40%) false-negative rate.[7,8] The high false-negative rate of FDG PET for small lesions seems to be related to respiratory and cardiac motion and the sequential nature for the acquisition of the PET and CT images when using a conventional PET/CT scanner.[9,10] Studies have demonstrated mild improvements of standardized uptake value (SUV) quantification in PET/CT of pulmonary nodules when respiratory motion correction, via external monitoring devices, is used.[11,12] Thus, motion-corrected PET reconstruction can potentially improve detection and characterization of pulmonary nodules.[13]

Hybrid PET/MR systems allow for simultaneous acquisition of PET and MR imaging. It has been shown that PET acquisition performed simultaneously with free-breathing radial T1-weighted MR acquisition has similar accuracy as PET/CT for FDG-avid lesions and lesions larger than 5 mm in size.[14] However, despite simultaneous acquisition of PET and MR, hybrid PET/MR has had low sensitivity for small pulmonary nodules that did not show FDG avidity. Thus, similar to PET/CT, conventional (without motion correction) simultaneous PET/MR remains limited for detection and characterization of small pulmonary nodules because of its inability to confidently detect FDG uptake in small lesions, which is likely related to motion blur and respiratory motion.

LUNG MOTION CORRECTION IN MAGNETIC RESONANCE/PET: PREVIOUS LIMITATIONS

Abdominal motion is still an outstanding concern for PET image reconstruction, particularly in the abdomen where rigid body approximations do not apply. Most of the motion correction algorithms previously used for PET image reconstruction rely on the use of retrospective corrections whereby the data are grouped according to the time of acquisition relative to the phase of the respiratory cycle (or any other motion of interest) as assessed by an additional motion tracking device

(usually a respiratory belt/cushion). In this setting, different segments from the list-mode data set, corresponding to different data acquisition times, will often be grouped together, regardless of whether the respiratory motion is periodic and/or the physiologic process stationary. As a result, the performance of such algorithms is highly variable as it depends strongly on the reproducibility of the respiratory motion throughout the examination. Unfortunately, studies have demonstrated that breathing motion varies considerably for healthy human controls and much more so for those individuals whereby lesion is present.[15] Consequently, respiratory motion correction via external tracking devices has limited effectiveness[13] and continues to be an area of active research in PET image reconstruction.[16–28] As a result, there is no standard for dealing with this challenge and the available methods are not often part of the clinical workflow for PET/CT and MR/PET examinations.

Retrospective Motion Correction for Magnetic Resonance/PET Data

Motion correction algorithms for MR/PET data were introduced shortly after the first system prototypes were delivered.[21,29,30] In the setting of MR/PET, the use of a simultaneous acquisition mode, whereby both MR and PET data are acquired at the same time, allows tracking the respiratory motion using MR signals (images or raw data). Use of the MR-based tracking information can be done prospectively and retrospectively. Retrospective approaches[21,31–34] are, conceptually, very similar to those previously used for PET/CT, whereby the data are, again, retrospectively reordered. Therefore, these algorithms are easy to implement but have limited effectiveness because they still suffer from some of the limitations stated earlier.

Prospective Motion Correction for Magnetic Resonance/PET Data

Prospective motion correction algorithms[26,27] rely on continuous information about the abdomen's deformation for the generation of motion fields that can then be used to dynamically distort the system matrix so that all the list-mode data can be intrinsically coregistered to a single-motion state or gate. As such, they do not require the respiratory motion to be periodic and can also be used during dynamic studies by simply binning the list-mode data for physiologically appropriate time windows. This approach is conceptually different from the methodology presented elsewhere in this volume. A brief description of its fundamental elements is, therefore, presented later.

In order to obtain a single-motion free PET reconstruction using this approach, the conventional straight-line model is extended by a motion component in which respiratory motion information is integrated within the PET system matrix. To achieve this, the expectation maximization algorithm

$$f^{k+1} = f^k \frac{1}{X^T 1} X^T \frac{g}{Xf^k} \tag{1}$$

is modified to

$$f^{k+1} = f^k \frac{1}{(XM)^T 1} (XM)^T \frac{g}{(XM) f^k} \tag{2}$$

where X represents the classic system matrix, M is the motion operator, f represents the desired image, and g contains the acquired emission data (ignoring attenuation and scatter correction for simplicity).

Fig. 1 illustrates the basic elements of a prospective elastic body motion correction approach. In this approach, list mode PET data are assigned system matrices according to the object's deformation at the time of their acquisition, as identified from MR-based signals (images or raw data). When motion is present, this is equivalent to elastic warping of the lines of response, thereby mapping the object to its original (reference) configuration. When the motion is periodic, this approach is functionally equivalent to a retrospective motion correction. However, when breathing is irregular, it still allows for correction of the PET counts as long as the configuration state of the abdomen can be readily identified from the MR imaging signal. Strategies for how to accomplish this last goal in a continuous fashion during a concurrent MR/PET examination are described later.

METHODS

All data were collected on a MR/PET scanner (Siemens Healthcare, GmbH, Germany). The system consists of a whole-body 3-T scanner, which is fitted with an MR imaging–compatible PET subsystem. The PET subsystem relies on an array of lutetium orthosilicate crystals coupled to avalanche photodiode scintillation detectors. The MR and PET subsystems are both electrically and mechanically independent, which allows for the acquisition of simultaneous data for both modalities. The MR subsystem has multichannel reception and is equipped with a whole-body gradient set capable of 45 mT/m (150 mT/m/s slew rate). The PET subsystem has 488 individual detectors (56 detector blocks, 8 detectors per block), which enable a nominal spatial resolution for the PET system of 4 × 4 × 4 mm in fully 3-dimensional mode.

Patients were recruited under an Institutional Review Board–approved protocol. All patients fasted for 4 hours before being administered a single intravenous injection of 18F-FDG. After resting in a quiet room, the patients underwent a standard-of-care, clinically prescribed, PET/CT examination and were then transported to the MR/PET facility to undergo a simultaneous MR/PET scan (on average 1.5 hours after the PET/CT examination).

Simultaneous MR/PET data were acquired using a 3-dimensional, radial T1-weighted sequence and list-mode data. The radial sequence sampled a set of parallel disks in the X-Y plane using golden angle increments for the radial views and standard phase encoding steps along the Z axis. This sequence, being self-navigated, provides the ability to order acquired views according to their position in the respiratory cycle. Images were then reconstructed using a compressed sensing algorithm to obtain an effective spatial and temporal resolution of 2 × 2 × 4 mm³ and 3 seconds, respectively. Each one of the acquired lines in k-space was time indexed in the PET list-mode data so that the temporal correspondence between acquired lines and lines of response could be accurately established. On reconstruction of the views ordered according to their phase on the respiratory cycle, a transformation matrix providing a nonelastic transformation (motion vectors) from each respiratory-ordered motion

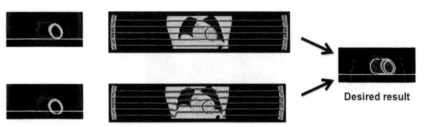

Desired result

Fig. 1. Prospective nonrigid body motion correction scheme. Motion at different phases of the respiratory cycle is incorporated via a modified system matrix with lines of response warped to account for the object's motion. The warping is specific to each motion state and does not require the object's displacement to be periodic.

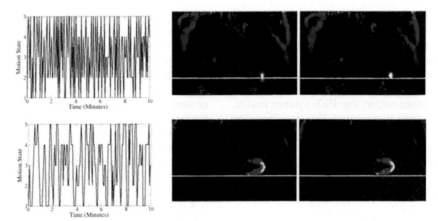

Fig. 2. Retrospective motion correction of nonrigid motion in MR/PET. Left: gate assignment trace. Center: uncorrected image. Right: reconstructed image based on a reordering of the PET list-mode data mode using the amplitude of the k-space center during a radial acquisition. Nonperiodic respiration compromises the effectives of the correction for the subject on the bottom row.

state to a reference state was calculated. These motion vectors then provide the prescription for distorting the lines of response as illustrated on **Fig. 1**.

RESULTS

The effects of stable respiratory motion on the performance of retrospective reordering are presented in **Fig. 2** where the MR-derived respiratory ordered signals are presented for 2 different subjects with vastly different respiratory cycles. As shown in **Fig. 2**, for the subject with the more regular respiratory cycle (top panel), the PET counts can be more uniformly distributed across 5 respiratory gates. As a result, motion correction leads to a measurable improvement in image quality. For the subject with the less regular respiratory cycle (bottom panel), the irregularity in the respiratory cycle leads to a large number of PET counts being mis-assigned; as a result, motion correction leads to nonsignificant improvements in image quality. These images illustrate the importance of conceptual advantage of prospective respiratory motion correction schemes

as well as the inherent disadvantages of retrospective motion correction approaches.

As mentioned earlier, lung nodule detection could be considerably improved by the use of the combined MR/PET platform. This point is illustrated in **Fig. 3** whereby PET images from a subject with suspected malignancy in the lung are presented. The subject's respiratory motion leads to significant blurring of the signal from the small lesion and as a result the assessed SUV could not warrant an aggressive course of action (left panel). On motion correction (center panel), the blurring is significantly reduced leading to both improved lesion localization as well as improved quantitative assessment of the tracer uptake (67% signal increase, rightmost panel).

Fig. 4 presents another example of improved small lesion detection using MR/PET-based motion correction. As in the previous case, the motion information was harnessed by retrospective reordering of the MR imaging data using the signal from the k-space center to synthesize 5 motion states. This time, despite the small lesion size, a sizable (>40%) improvement in SUV can be observed after

Fig. 3. Prospective elastic motion correction in MR/PET. Left: uncorrected image. Center: reconstructed image based on a dynamic motion model derived from a volumetric radial data set with at time resolution of 1 second. Right: plot of signal along the vertical line in the leftmost image demonstrating increased signal (67%) for the lung lesion as a result of motion correction.

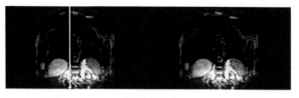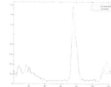

Fig. 4. Another example of prospective elastic motion correction in the lung. Left: uncorrected image. Center: reconstructed image based on a dynamic motion model derived from a volumetric radial data set with at time resolution of 1 second. Right: plot of signal along the vertical line in the leftmost image demonstrating increased signal (40%) for the lung lesion as a result of motion correction.

the blurring in the images is ameliorated through the use of the motion correction algorithm.

DISCUSSION

The development of the PET/CT platform in the late 1990s clearly illustrated the clinical throughput and diagnostic advantages of combining image modalities that have inherently complementary information.[35] The developmental motivation for the PET/CT platform, though simple in concept, led to the widespread adoption of the PET/CT technology over conventional PET-only scans. Over the years, however, the sequential nature of the PET and CT acquisitions, and the need to keep the CT acquisition short, have not allowed for a true synergistic interaction between PET/CT's component modalities in which the combined platform allows the generation of better images than those that could be individually acquired with each modality on its own.

MR/PET is the first hybrid-imaging platform whereby the images that could be generated for each of its component modalities could, in principle, be of improved quality when the salient features for the individual imaging modalities are combined in a synergistic fashion. In MR/PET this is due by and large to the simultaneous nature of the acquisition, which allows collecting information about the imaged volume with intrinsic temporal and spatial colocalization. Such colocalization allows exploiting the differences in the acquisition physics and geometry to improve image quality. One of the most readily immediate advantages of MR/PET derives from MR's speed of acquisition and customizable acquisition strategies. Specifically, by rapidly acquiring images in complete synchrony with the detection of PET events information about the geometric configuration of the imaged volume could be used in near real time to compensate for the deleterious effects of abdominal motion. The aforementioned examples illustrated that the gains to be had from such capabilities can be harnessed without an inherent burden to the overall data acquisition time.

Self-navigated imaging sequences such as the one used in the aforementioned examples represent an ideal vehicle for the integration of motion correction capabilities in a combine MR/PET scan. There are, however, other options to gather motion information from the MR imaging signal that could potentially lead to more comprehensive and robust means to assess the geometric changes in the imaged volume.[36] Although such methods are still in early development, initial results indicate that they have intrinsic advantages for the assessment irregular and nonstationary motion. Overall, the technical developments and experimental results shown to date indicate that PET motion correction is likely to be one of the most robust and salient features of the MR/PET platform. Initial clinical experience (as illustrated earlier) indicates that there are considerable benefits to be gained from such methodology with very minimal (if at all) disruption to patient workflow. At the time of this writing, commercial prototypes for approaches similar to the one presented here have been in active evaluation by equipment manufacturers, which suggests that such methodology will quickly become part of the standard workflow for MR/PET examinations of the abdomen.

REFERENCES

1. Laymon CM, Bowsher JE. Anomaly detection and artifact recovery in pet attenuation-correction images using the likelihood function. IEEE J Sel Top Signal Process 2013;7(1).

2. Knoll F, Koesters T, Otazo R, et al. Joint reconstruction of simultaneously acquired MR-PET data with multi sensor compressed sensing based on a joint sparsity constraint. EJNMMI Phys 2014; 1(Suppl 1):A26.

3. Girvin F, Ko JP. Pulmonary nodules: detection, assessment, and CAD. AJR Am J Roentgenol 2008;191(4):1057–69.

4. Benjamin MS, Drucker EA, McLoud TC, et al. Small pulmonary nodules: detection at chest CT and outcome. Radiology 2003;226(2):489–93.

5. Cistaro A, Lopci E, Gastaldo L, et al. The role of 18F-FDG PET/CT in the metabolic characterization of lung nodules in pediatric patients with bone sarcoma. Pediatr Blood Cancer 2012;59(7): 1206–10.

6. Schillaci O, Travascio L, Bolacchi F, et al. Accuracy of early and delayed FDG PET-CT and of contrast-enhanced CT in the evaluation of lung nodules: a preliminary study on 30 patients. Radiol Med 2009; 114(6):890–906.

7. Mayerhoefer ME, Prosch H, Herold CJ, et al. Assessment of pulmonary melanoma metastases with 18F-FDG PET/CT: which PET-negative patients require additional tests for definitive staging? Eur Radiol 2012;22(11):2451–7.

8. Bamba Y, Itabashi M, Kameoka S. Value of PET/CT imaging for diagnosing pulmonary metastasis of colorectal cancer. Hepatogastroenterology 2011; 58(112):1972–4.

9. Nomori H, Watanabe K, Ohtsuka T, et al. Evaluation of F-18 fluorodeoxyglucose (FDG) PET scanning for pulmonary nodules less than 3 cm in diameter, with special reference to the CT images. Lung Cancer 2004;45(1):19–27.

10. Watanabe K, Nomori H, Ohtsuka T, et al. False negative cases of F-18 fluorodeoxyglucose-positron emission tomography (FDG-PET) imaging in small lung cancer less than 3 cm in size. Nihon Kokyuki Gakkai Zasshi 2004;42(9):787–93 [in Japanese].

11. Apostolova I, Wiemker R, Paulus T, et al. Combined correction of recovery effect and motion blur for SUV quantification of solitary pulmonary nodules in FDG PET/CT. Eur Radiol 2010;20(8): 1868–77.

12. Werner MK, Parker JA, Kolodny GM, et al. Respiratory gating enhances imaging of pulmonary nodules and measurement of tracer uptake in FDG PET/CT. AJR Am J Roentgenol 2009;193(6): 1640–5.

13. Liu C, Pierce LA 2nd, Alessio AM, et al. The impact of respiratory motion on tumor quantification and delineation in static PET/CT imaging. Phys Med Biol 2009;54(24):7345–62.

14. Chandarana H, Heacock L, Rakheja R, et al. Pulmonary nodules in patients with primary malignancy: comparison of hybrid PET/MR and PET/CT imaging. Radiology 2013;268(3): 874–81.

15. Shirato H, Suzuki K, Sharp GC, et al. Speed and amplitude of lung tumor motion precisely detected in four-dimensional setup and in real-time tumor-tracking radiotherapy. Int J Radiat Oncol Biol Phys 2006;64(4):1229–36.

16. Yu Y, Chan C, Ma T, et al. Event-by-event continuous respiratory motion correction for dynamic PET imaging. J Nucl Med 2016;57(7): 1084–90.

17. Manber R, Thielemans K, Hutton BF, et al. Practical PET respiratory motion correction in clinical PET/MR. J Nucl Med 2015;56(6):890–6.

18. Fayad H, Schmidt H, Wuerslin C, et al. Reconstruction-incorporated respiratory motion correction in clinical simultaneous PET/MR imaging for oncology applications. J Nucl Med 2015;56(6): 884–9.

19. Balfour DR, Marsden PK, Polycarpou I, et al. Respiratory motion correction of PET using MR-constrained PET-PET registration. Biomed Eng Online 2015;14(1):85.

20. Manber R, Thielemans K, Hutton B, et al. Initial evaluation of a practical PET respiratory motion correction method in clinical simultaneous PET/MRI. EJNMMI Phys 2014;1(Suppl 1):A40.

21. Wurslin C, Schmidt H, Martirosian P, et al. Respiratory motion correction in oncologic PET using T1-weighted MR imaging on a simultaneous whole-body PET/MR system. J Nucl Med 2013;54(3): 464–71.

22. Chan C, Jin X, Fung EK, et al. Event-by-event respiratory motion correction for PET with 3D internal-1D external motion correlation. Med Phys 2013;40(11): 112507.

23. Liu C, Alessio AM, Kinahan PE. Respiratory motion correction for quantitative PET/CT using all detected events with internal-external motion correlation. Med Phys 2011;38(5):2715–23.

24. Bai W, Brady M. Motion correction and attenuation correction for respiratory gated PET images. IEEE Trans Med Imaging 2011;30(2):351–65.

25. Dawood M, Kosters T, Fieseler M, et al. Motion correction in respiratory gated cardiac PET/CT using multi-scale optical flow. Med Image Comput Comput Assist Interv 2008;11(Pt 2):155–62.

26. Lamare F, Ledesma Carbayo MJ, Cresson T, et al. List-mode-based reconstruction for respiratory motion correction in PET using non-rigid body transformations. Phys Med Biol 2007;52(17): 5187–204.

27. Lamare F, Cresson T, Savean J, et al. Respiratory motion correction for PET oncology applications using affine transformation of list mode data. Phys Med Biol 2007;52(1):121–40.

28. Dawood M, Lang N, Jiang X, et al. Lung motion correction on respiratory gated 3-D PET/CT images. IEEE Trans Med Imaging 2006;25(4): 476–85.

29. Catana C. Motion correction options in PET/MRI. Semin Nucl Med 2015;45(3):212–23.

30. Catana C, Benner T, van der Kouwe A, et al. MRI-assisted PET motion correction for neurologic studies

in an integrated MR-PET scanner. J Nucl Med 2011;
52(1):154–61.

31. Guerin B, Cho S, Chun SY, et al. Nonrigid PET motion compensation in the lower abdomen using simultaneous tagged-MRI and PET imaging. Med Phys 2011;38(6):3025–38.

32. Grimm R, Furst S, Souvatzoglou M, et al. Self-gated MRI motion modeling for respiratory motion compensation in integrated PET/MRI. Med Image Anal 2015;19(1):110–20.

33. Grimm R, Furst S, Dregely I, et al. Self-gated radial MRI for respiratory motion compensation on hybrid PET/MR systems. Med Image Comput Comput Assist Interv 2013;16(Pt 3):17–24.

34. Chun SY, Reese TG, Ouyang J, et al. MRI-based nonrigid motion correction in simultaneous PET/MRI. J Nucl Med 2012;53(8):1284–91.

35. Kinahan PE, Townsend DW, Beyer T, et al. Attenuation correction for a combined 3D PET/CT scanner. Med Phys 1998;25(10):2046–53.

36. Koesters T, Brown R, Zhao T, et al. Motion correcting complete MR/PET exams via pilot tone navigators. Annual Meeting of the International Society for Magnetic Resonance in Medicine. Singapore, May 7-13, 2016.

Practical Considerations for Clinical PET/MR Imaging

Samuel Galgano, MD[a], Zachary Viets, MD[b],
Kathryn Fowler, MD[b], Lael Gore, CNMT, RT[a],
John V. Thomas, MD[a], Michelle McNamara, MD[a],
Jonathan McConathy, MD, PhD[a],*

KEYWORDS

- PET/MR imaging • Whole-body PET/MR imaging • Oncologic imaging • PET/MR imaging protocols
- FDG-PET

KEY POINTS

- PET/MR imaging is in routine clinical use at multiple sites in the United States, Europe, and Asia.
- Clinical PET/MR imaging protocols include whole-body (WB) PET/MR imaging, regional PET/MR imaging, and a combination of WB and regional PET/MR imaging.
- Most oncologic PET/MR imaging studies include WB standard-of-care PET as well as regional standard-of-care MR imaging.
- PET acquisition and MR imaging sequences should be tailored to the clinical question, to maximize efficiency, and minimize the overall image acquisition time.

WORKFLOW, PROTOCOLLING, REPORTING AND BILLING

The workflow for clinical PET/MR imaging studies has similarities to PET/computed tomography (CT) and MR imaging studies but requires coordination at the scheduling, technologist, and interpreting physician levels, which may not exist initially. As few technologists, radiologist, and nuclear medicine physicians have trained in the era of PET/MR imaging, it is often necessary to have personnel with PET expertise to closely work with those with MR imaging expertise and to cross-train in the modality they are less familiar with. Many programs begin by performing crossover studies with patients undergoing clinical PET/CT studies then immediately afterward undergoing PET/MR imaging studies with the same radiopharmaceutical administration. An example of a clinical PET/MR imaging workflow is shown schematically in **Fig. 1**.

There are some considerations with clinical PET/MR imaging studies that differ from PET/CT and MR imaging. Many PET/MR imaging studies involve standard-of-care PET and MR imaging studies that must be precertified. The need for precertification can slow the scheduling of PET/MR imaging studies compared with PET/CT or MR imaging studies, which in turn may be frustrating to referring physicians and patients. In some clinical

This article originally appeared in *Magnetic Resonance Imaging Clinics*, Volume 25, Issue 2, May 2017.

Dr J. McConathy is a consultant for Siemens Healthcare, GE Healthcare, Blue Earth Diagnostics, and Eli Lilly/ Avid. Drs S. Galgano, Z. Viets, K. Fowler, L. Gore, J.V. Thomas, and M. McNamara have nothing to disclose.

[a] Department of Radiology, University of Alabama at Birmingham (UAB), 619 19th Street South, Birmingham, AL 35249, USA; [b] Department of Radiology, Washington University in St Louis, 510 South Kingshighway Boulevard, St. Louis, MO 63110, USA

* Corresponding author. Division of Molecular Imaging and Therapeutics, 619 19th Street, Jefferson Tower 773, Birmingham, AL 35249.

E-mail address: jmcconathy@uabmc.edu

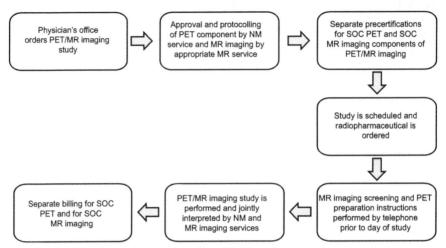

Fig. 1. Example of a clinical PET/MR imaging workflow. SOC, standard of care.

practices, radiology schedulers perform the pre-certification, which can reduce the burden on the referring physician's office. Another consideration is that some patients will not be able to complete the PET/MR imaging examination because of the length of the study and/or claustrophobia. Ideally, PET/CT would be available as a backup so that the PET radiopharmaceutical administration will not be wasted and expose the patient to radiation without providing diagnostic information.

Most institutions select patients with standard-of-care indications for both PET and MR imaging for evaluation through PET/MR imaging studies. For oncology, the protocol often consists of a whole-body (WB) PET along with WB-MR imaging for staging and a regional diagnostic MR imaging examination for assessment of the primary tumor and/or regional nodal staging. As with PET/CT, the WB component is typically varied depending on the type and location of the tumor with typical WB coverage from skull base to midthigh (most solid tumors), skull vertex to midthigh (eg, head and neck cancers), skull vertex to knee (eg, multiple myeloma, some melanomas), or skull vertex to toes (eg, some melanomas and malignancies of the lower extremities). For brain and cardiac PET/MR imaging studies, both the PET and the MR imaging acquisitions are typically regional only without a WB component. This approach reduces the overall time required for patient imaging (1 session instead of 2), allows simultaneous review of both PET and MR imaging studies by the interpreting physicians, and can streamline the diagnostic imaging process. For some patients, PET/MR imaging is performed for standard-of-care PET indications without a diagnostic MR imaging component. A common reason to perform PET/MR imaging without a diagnostic MR imaging

examination is for dose reduction in children and young adults by replacing WB CT with MR imaging for attenuation correction (AC) and anatomic localization.

The PET protocol for simultaneous PET/MR imaging studies involves selecting the appropriate PET tracer for the indication as well as the region to be covered by PET (limited, skull base to midthigh, WB). **Table 1** provides a list of the Food and Drug Administration (FDA)–approved PET tracers and their primary clinical applications. Most PET studies in the United States are for oncologic indications and use the glucose analogue 2-deoxy-2-[^{18}F]fluoro-D-glucose ([^{18}F] FDG). The MR imaging protocol for simultaneous PET/MR imaging involves the MR imaging sequences for the WB-PET/MR imaging portion of the study and/or the protocol for the regional MR imaging protocol. For PET/MR imaging studies that include a diagnostic MR imaging component, the protocol is typically based on the same protocol used for MR imaging–only examinations, although some sequences may be omitted or adapted to reduce the total amount of time required for the PET/MR imaging examination. Depending on the training of those involved, the PET protocolling may be done by nuclear medicine, whereas the MR imaging protocolling is typically done by the appropriate radiology subspecialty.

The interpretation of PET/MR imaging requires fusion of PET with multiple MR imaging sequences, and several commercially available software packages are suitable for this purpose. However, some software packages that work well for PET/CT are not readily adapted to PET/MR imaging because of the need to fuse the PET images with mutli-planar, multi-sequence MR

Table 1
Food and Drug Administration–approved PET tracers (2016)

PET Tracer	Primary Clinical Applications
[^{13}N]Ammonia	Myocardial perfusion
[^{11}C]Choline chloride	Detection and staging of recurrent prostate cancer
[^{18}F]FDG	Cancer diagnosis, staging and treatment response Neuroimaging for epilepsy and dementia Cardiac imaging for myocardial viability Inflammation and infection
[^{68}Ga]DOTATATE	Somatostatin-receptor positive tumors, especially neuroendocrine tumors
[^{18}F]Florbetaben	Detection of brain amyloid
[^{18}F]Florbetapir	Detection of brain amyloid
[^{18}F]Fluciclovine	Detection and staging of recurrent prostate cancer
[^{18}F]Flutemetamol	Detection of brain amyloid
[^{82}Rb]Rubidium chloride	Myocardial perfusion
Sodium [^{18}F]fluoride	Skeletal scintigraphy for osseous metastases

imaging acquisitions and to work with relatively large numbers of image series. Local practice pattern will determine how PET/MR imaging studies are interpreted. At some institutions, the PET portion of the study is read by nuclear medicine and the diagnostic MR imaging portion is read by the appropriate radiology subspecialty. This strategy can provide the highest level of subspecialty expertise for each component of the study but requires coordination and discussion before issuing the PET/MR imaging report. Alternatively, a single reader with appropriate training may read the entire study. The Society of Nuclear Medicine and Molecular Imaging and the American College of Radiology (ACR) are in the process of developing practice standards for interpreting

PET/MR imaging studies and have issued guidelines for neuroimaging with PET/MR imaging.[1]

Reporting of PET/MR imaging studies that include standard-of-care PET and diagnostic regional MR imaging can be reported separately or as a single integrated report. Some institutions use separate reports for the PET and MR imaging components to facilitate billing. When separate reporting is performed, the WB MR imaging findings are typically included with the PET report in a similar fashion to the CT portion of PET/CT studies. The findings should be harmonized if separate reports are issued, and the PET and MR imaging reports should cross-reference each other for clarity in the medical record and for the ordering physician. Billing in the United States is based on the appropriate PET-only *Current Procedural Terminology* (*CPT*) code (78811, 78112, 78813) and MR imaging *CPT* codes. Currently, no PET/MR imaging–specific *CPT* codes are available as there are for PET/CT. Although systematic data regarding billing and reimbursement for PET/MR imaging are not available, most centers performing clinical PET/MR imaging report similar reimbursement for PET/MR imaging as for their PET/CT and MR imaging studies.

MR IMAGING AND RADIATION SAFETY

The location and facilities housing a PET/MR imaging scanner should follow institutional and national guidelines regarding MR imaging and radiation safety, which includes adherence to the MR imaging zones I to IV to ensure patient safety.[2] The waiting room for the PET/MR imaging scanner should follow guidelines to be an MR imaging zone I with patient prescreening taking place in MR imaging zone II. Patients undergoing PET/MR imaging should be routinely prescreened before entering MR imaging zones III and IV by appropriately qualified and trained personnel. Only patients deemed safe to undergo MR imaging should be allowed into zones III and IV, always with supervision by the technologists. Because personnel working in PET/CT centers may not be as familiar with MR imaging safety guidelines as MR imaging technologists, particular care should be taken to ensure the use of MR–compatible patient monitoring devices to avoid the risk of metallic projectiles in the PET/MR suite.

Implantable devices are a common issue in regard to MR imaging safety. At this time, all FDA-approved PET/MR imaging scanners operate at 3 Tesla (T). At the authors' institution, patients are required to provide documentation of the exact model and make of any implantable devices or to have documentation available in their medical records. Once the specific device is identified, information from the manufacturer and from online resources, such as MRIsafety.com, is available to determine safety in a 3-T magnetic field. Implanted pacemakers and automatic implantable cardioverter-defibrillators (AICDs) are historically a general contraindication to MR imaging. However, a growing body of research has demonstrated safety of certain implanted cardiac devices in MR imaging scanners.[3,4] In regard to PET/MR imaging, a major issue remains that implanted cardiac device safety is predominantly demonstrated in 1.5-T MR,[5] and there may be insufficient evidence for some devices to support safety in a 3-T MR imaging scanner.

Several MR imaging and PET safety concerns remain unique to women, the most common relating to pregnancy and lactation. Although MR imaging has been deemed safe during pregnancy, the current "ACR Guidance Document on MR Safe Practices"[2] states that MR imaging should only be considered in pregnant women if other imaging modalities without ionizing radiation will not provide appropriate clinical information, the information is likely to alter patient care, and the examination cannot be delayed until after pregnancy. It is the authors' institutional policy to obtain informed consent from any patient undergoing MR imaging while pregnant regarding the theoretic risks and benefits of the MR imaging procedure. Additionally, the radiation risks during pregnancy and potential benefit from the PET study should be discussed with the referring physician and patients, and PET/MR imaging may be preferable for pregnant patients because of the lack of additional radiation dose from CT. For young women with intrauterine devices, standard prescreening protocols should be undertaken as described earlier.

Gadolinium-based contrast is generally considered a very safe contrast medium, with very few adverse reactions observed. However, the administration of gadolinium-based contrast media to patients with severe chronic renal disease (glomerular filtration rate <30), acute kidney injury, and pregnant patients is contraindicated. Standard institutional policies should be undertaken to screen for renal dysfunction in patients at high risk to minimize the risk of the development of nephrogenic systemic fibrosis. Several studies have demonstrated minimal excretion of gadolinium into breast milk, and the ACR "Manual on Contrast Media"[6] deems MR imaging with gadolinium-based contrast safe for breastfeeding women without cessation of lactation for any period of time. However, it is often necessary to temporarily interrupt breastfeeding to limit the infant's effective dose from the PET tracer to less than 1 mSv (100 mrem). The length of cessation will depend on the PET tracer and the amount of activity administered and should meet federal, state, and institutional regulations and policy.

A unique MR imaging safety concern to PET/MR imaging is the ability to shield and administer intravenous agents (radiopharmaceuticals and contrast) in an MR imaging–compatible fashion. Care should be undertaken so that all shielding material is MR imaging compatible, and there are reports of lead shielding moving under the influence of a strong magnetic field.[7] Tungsten-based MR imaging–compatible syringe shields have been developed for use in the PET/MR imaging environment and are commercially available. Similarly, cardiac monitoring systems and automated injectors for PET radiopharmaceuticals must be MR imaging compatible. The areas for storing and handling PET radiopharmaceuticals should be configured in accordance with institutional, state, and national guidelines and does not differ from the setup used for a PET/CT suite. Standard technologist PET radiation safety protocols should be undertaken in accordance with state and national guidelines and also do not differ from PET/CT.

PET/MR imaging offers the advantage of performing the anatomic imaging portion of the examination without ionizing radiation. Although ionizing radiation from the radiopharmaceutical used for PET is inevitable, previous studies have demonstrated that up to 70% of the radiation dose of a PET/CT is due to the CT dose,[8–12] although the CT dose can be lowered depending on the acquisition technique. The high sensitivity of current PET/MR imaging systems as well as the potential to acquire PET data for a longer period of time during MR imaging sequence acquisition have the potential to reduce the radiation dose to patients related to the radiopharmaceutical.[13,14]

WHOLE-BODY PET/MR IMAGING ACQUISITION

This section focuses on WB protocols designed for simultaneous PET/MR imaging, although many of the same considerations apply to sequential PET/MR imaging systems. The primary clinical use of WB PET/MR imaging is currently for cancer staging; thus, oncologic PET/MR imaging is the focus of this section. Other applications, such as evaluating for systemic infectious and inflammatory processes, are relevant as well but are less commonly performed in routine clinical practice. There is a lack of clear consensus among PET/MR imaging users regarding a core WB protocol, and no large studies comparing the diagnostic accuracy of different WB MR imaging protocols used with PET/MR imaging for specific clinical applications have been published.

Comparison of Whole-Body PET/MR Imaging and PET/Computed Tomography Protocols

There are several important differences between PET/CT and PET/MR for WB imaging. With PET/CT, typically a low-dose CT scan is acquired for anatomic localization and AC, followed by the PET acquisition. At some institutions, diagnostic CT examinations with intravenous contrast may be performed as well. The technologist must manipulate either the PET or CT field of view (FOV) to ensure proper alignment and adhesion regarding start/stop times and locations. A relatively new technology in PET/CT called continuous bed motion allows technologists to prescribe both FOV simultaneously and has the potential to decrease scan time and radiation dose.[15] Because PET/CT is a sequential image acquisition, PET/CT motion artifacts and misregistration can occur.[16] WB-PET/MR acquisition requires the technologist to accurately place body coils before beginning the study. Next, a WB localizer scan is needed for anatomic layout and PET bed placement. Finally, desired MR sequences are assigned to each PET bed. Each bed contains its own MRAC map scan as well as any additional MR imaging sequences in the protocol. An example of console settings for a WB PET/MR imaging study is shown in **Fig. 2.**

Simultaneous PET/MR facilitates consistent spatial and temporal correspondence between the PET and MR imaging acquisitions and can minimize misregistration. In the chest and abdomen, free-breathing MR sequences and/or respiratory gating techniques can be used to reduce misregistration between PET and MR imaging data.[17,18] However, misregistration can still occur with simultaneous acquisition, which can lead to AC artifacts and mis-localization of PET findings. MR imaging often uses breath holds for motion-free imaging, whereas PET acquisitions take too long to be acquired during a single breath hold. This difference in image collection commonly leads to misregistration errors in chest and abdominal imaging. An example of the type of motion artifact and misregistration that can occur with PET acquisition during breath-hold MR imaging is shown in **Fig. 3.** Respiratory gating and tracker programs that use liver position to engage acquisition can improve registration of the PET and MR imaging data in the lower chest and upper abdomen and decrease blurring of the PET data.[19–21]

Currently, simultaneous acquisition PET/MR scanners in clinical use have a bore diameter of 60 cm to accommodate an integrated PET ring, which is substantially less than the typical 70 cm diameter found in PET/CT and traditional MR imaging. The smaller bore can present a unique challenge to even an average body habitus after coil placement and gantry advancement. Patients who have been able to undergo

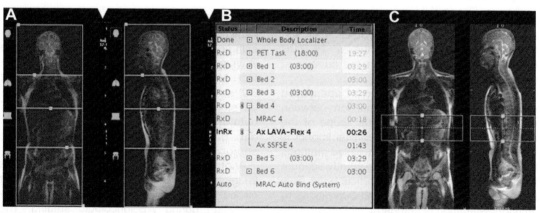

Fig. 2. Example of console for WB PET/MR imaging acquisition. (*A*) Visual inspection ensures 3-plane MR imaging localizer falls within PET bed parameters (*red guidelines right of localizer, white arrowhead*) and all anatomy is accounted for. Head, chest, abdomen, and pelvis drag bars are then used to differentiate anatomy and assign appropriate segmentation algorithms. (*B*) A prescription box displaying MR sequences within each PET bed. Time per sequence as well as the total time per bed are displayed. The sequences within PET bed 4 are shown midprescription. (*C*) The MR prescription within PET bed 4. Because MR sequences are linked to corresponding PET beds at isocenter, copy and paste can be used to assign the exact same MR prescription to each PET bed. This method ensures identical parameters for similar sequences enabling postprocessing editing for contiguous review. LAVA-Flex and SSFSE sequences are from GE Healthcare (Milwaukee, WI).

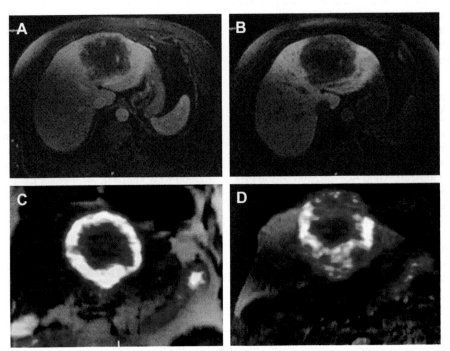

Fig. 3. Selected MR imaging and FDG-PET/MR images in a patient with liver metastases from colon cancer. Representative dynamic axial T1-weighted MR images obtained after the administration of a hepatobiliary MR contrast agent, gadoxetate disodium, in the venous phase (*A*) and the hepatobiliary phase (*B*) show a large metastasis in the left hepatic lobe, which is centrally necrotic. The hepatobiliary phase images in panel (*B*) better define the tumor margins and are useful for detecting small metastases as hypointense lesions because of the increasing enhancement of liver during the hepatobiliary phase. The fused coronal T2-weighted image (*C*) demonstrated high FDG uptake in the periphery of the tumor and good alignment between the MR imaging and PET without motion artifact as both were acquired during free breathing. The fused coronal T1-weighted hepatobiliary phase postcontrast image (*D*) shows significant motion artifact and misregistration due to PET acquisition during the multiple breath holds performed for dynamic postcontrast MR imaging. This type of motion artifact shown in panel (*D*) can be corrected with respiratory gating if accurate coregistration of PET with the postcontrast MR imaging is required.

traditional MR imaging–only studies may find themselves unable to continue a PET/MR because of the restriction from the number of coils required in WB scanning.

Although thorough discussion of attenuation correction methods and comparison between CTAC and MRAC is beyond the scope of the article, a brief mention of the clinical impact is warranted. MRAC segmentation-based methods for clinical WB imaging do not currently account for the attenuation effects of cortical bone. This lack of representation of cortical bone leads to an underestimation of standardized uptake value (SUV) for osseous lesions by an average of 11% and up to 16% for sclerotic spine lesions.[22] The impact on clinical staging of osseous metastases in uncertain, and many investigators have demonstrated no difference in detection and in some instances improved visual conspicuity of PET/MR imaging findings when compared with PET/CT.[23–25] The added value of improved depiction of marrow replacing lesions on MR imaging compared with CT should also be factored in when considering the clinical impact of imperfect MRAC. However, direct comparison of SUVs between PET/MR imaging and PET/CT studies is not possible; comparison of PET data acquired on PET/MR imaging with normal data bases acquired with PET/CT may not be appropriate.

Another major difference between PET/MR imaging and PET/CT with potential resultant clinical impact is that of pulmonary nodule detection during WB oncologic staging. The ability of most MR sequences to depict small pulmonary nodules is markedly limited because of respiratory motion, low proton density, and susceptibility artifact related to air within lung tissues. The detection rates for pulmonary nodules range from 36% to 96% depending on the used MR sequence and the size of the pulmonary nodules.[26–30] Which sequences provide greatest sensitivity for detection remains controversial; turbo spin echo (TSE) and triggered short-tau inversion recovery (STIR) images provided greatest sensitivity in one study, whereas in another study 3-dimensional (3D) gradient echo images were most accurate. Overall, in studies comparing staging accuracy of MR imaging with CT for determining surgical candidacy in patients with lung cancer, MR provided similar results.[31–33] However, for purposes of WB staging, a diagnostic chest CT may be warranted to complement the PET/MR imaging examination if detecting subcentimeter pulmonary nodules will alter patient management.

Sequences

The total acquisition time is an important consideration both in terms of patients' ability to tolerate the study and for patient throughput. Several protocols have been proposed with a variety of MR imaging sequences, and the need for clinically tailored approaches is a recurrent theme.[23,34–36] A core component of MR imaging acquisitions for PET/MR imaging is a sequence for MRAC. This topic is discussed in greater detail in Yasheng Chen and Hongyu An's article, "Attenuation Correction of PET/MR Imaging," in this issue. Both vendors with commercially available simultaneous PET/MR scanners currently use similar MRAC approaches in clinical practice. A 2-point Dixon sequence separates 3D spoiled gradient echo images into water-only and fat-only images used to segment tissues into 4 components: air, lung, fat, and soft tissues.[37] In addition to the MRAC provided with the Dixon sequence, images with fat weighting, water weighting, in-phase, and opposed-phase sequences are generated and can be fused with the PET data for review. An example of the Dixon-derived WB MR imaging sequences is shown in **Fig. 4**.

The most basic WB PET/MR protocol typically consists of a 2- to 3-minute PET bed acquisition along with accompanying MR sequences. When prescribed, these sequences originate from the PET bed iso-center because of the PET-MR FOV relationship. MRAC sequences are acquired first to generate an MR-based AC map. While generally of lower spatial resolution than typical diagnostic MR imaging sequences, these images are acquired with isotropic voxels allowing for reconstructions in any plane without image blurring or stair stepping artifact. These MRAC sequences are acquired rapidly (on the order of 20 seconds per bed position) and, thus, do not contribute greatly to the overall length of PET/MR imaging studies.

T2-weighted (T2W) sequences are useful for illustrating both normal anatomy and pathological processes, and many WB MR imaging sequences use free-breathing T2 axial and/or coronal sequences (eg, single shot techniques) as core WB imaging sequences for PET/MR imaging. An example of a coronal WB T2 single shot image is shown in **Fig. 4**, and the enhanced soft-tissue contrast and resolution compared with the Dixon sequences can be useful for lesion characterization. Other T2W sequences include multi-breath hold and navigated techniques such as T2 fat-suppressed images in place of or in addition to single shot techniques. The single shot technique uses one pulse excitation to produce many refocused echoes that fill the center of k-space in sub-seconds. These sequences produce robust T2 weighting, can acquire large FOVs in short periods of time, and are free from motion artifact. However, there may be offset between slices due to respiratory motion throughout the acquisition. Navigated sequences can use diaphragmatic motion or external bellows to trigger acquisition. These sequences tend to take longer depending on the efficiency of capturing either end-expiration or end-inspiration. Small FOV high-resolution T2W imaging also forms the basis for local staging of many pelvic tumors, including cervical cancer and prostate cancer.

T1-weighted (T1W) sequences may be acquired and are used primarily for anatomic detail and may be particularly valuable for assessing lesions affecting mineralized bone. T1W WB gadolinium-based contrast-enhanced imaging may be useful for certain oncologic indications, such as multiple myeloma, whereby sensitivity for lesion detection is increased.[38] LAVA-Flex (similar to Dixon VIBE) is a T1W 3D dual-echo techniques can be used to provide in-phase, out-of-phase, fat, and water-separated images in less than a minute. This sequence provides definitive water and fat separation over large inhomogeneous FOVs that would hinder many fat-suppression techniques. Depending on anatomy and parameters, 3D T1W images can be acquired rapidly allowing for breath holding (typically on the order of 20 seconds or less).

Diffusion-weighted imaging (DWI) provides a surrogate measure of cellular density by exploiting the impedance of the Brownian motion of water molecules in tissues of different cellularity and composition. It is a T2-based image acquired at multiple gradients (b values) with the slope of the diffusion data converted into an apparent diffusion coefficient (ADC) map showing tissues of high cellularity as bright on DWI and dark on ADC. ADC values have been shown to inversely

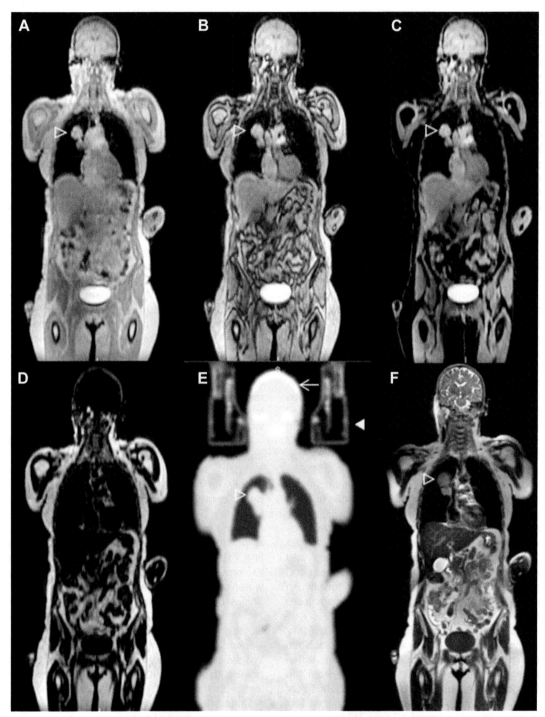

Fig. 4. Dixon sequences for MR-based attenuation correction in a patient undergoing initial staging of non–small cell lung cancer. The primary tumor is indicated with an open arrowhead. The MR images derived from the Dixon sequence are shown: in phase (A), opposed phase (B), water (C), and fat (D) and can be used for anatomic localization as shown in Fig. 4. A coronal MR-derived AC map image is shown in panel (E), which segments tissues into air, lung, fat and soft tissue throughout the body. In the head, the location of cortical bone is estimated and included in this AC map (white arrow). Additionally, the head coil is represented in the AC map (white arrowhead). For comparison, a WB T2-weighted single-shot fast-spine echo image is also shown (F).

correlate with FDG uptake in many but not all tumor histologies.[39–42] DWI may be acquired as a free-breathing or navigated sequence and can also be gated to correct for motion. DWI is useful as an adjunct for diagnosis in dedicated MR acquisitions; however, its added value over FDG in WB-PET/MR imaging remains controversial and difficult to balance against the time penalty of acquiring DWI at each station.[43,44] DWI may be more valuable when using PET tracers other than FDG that provide distinct biological information, such as hypoxia, apoptosis, or receptor status.

Tailoring PET/MR Imaging to the Clinical Application

The clinical indication and the goal of the PET/MR imaging examination are important considerations when selecting the WB protocol. For some PET/MR imaging studies, such neuroimaging for primary brain tumors, dementia, or epilepsy, and myocardial perfusion imaging, no WB study is indicated. In contrast, most PET/MR imaging studies for cancer will include WB staging, as the detection of unsuspected regional and distant metastases is one of the primary strengths of FDG-PET and other oncologic PET tracers. From a study length perspective, the most efficient WB-PET/MR imaging protocol will match the time required for WB-MR imaging sequence acquisition to the length of PET acquisition at each bed position, which is typically on the order of 2 to 3 minutes. However, in some cases additional MR imaging sequences, such as DWI, requiring longer acquisition times may be desirable. The overall length of the WB and regional MR imaging components (if any) of the examination must be considered to avoid an excessively lengthy study time. To be considered competitive against PET/CT, WB scan times would ideally be completed within 30 minutes or less and include MR sequences best suited to the specific clinical question. In general, a total examination time for combined WB and regional PET/MR imaging studies is 60 minutes or less of total image acquisition time.

In many cases, attenuation correction of the PET data and the anatomic localization of the PET findings on MRAC images are sufficient for clinical WB-PET/MR imaging staging examinations. In this scenario, the WB-MR imaging sequences are acting as a substitute for the CT images of a PET/CT study; data suggest that the Dixon sequences for MRAC are noninferior to PET/CT in terms of localizing PET findings when performing WB staging with FDG-PET in oncology.[45] An example of using Dixon sequences for anatomic localization in a patient with non–small cell lung

cancer is shown in **Fig. 5**. This strategy is most likely to be effective in malignancies that have uniformly high uptake of the PET tracer, such as FDG in aggressive lymphomas, whereby PET-negative sites of viable malignancy are unlikely.[46,47] Because of the short acquisition time for the Dixon MRAC sequence, additional MR imaging sequences can be used during the 2- to 3-minute PET acquisition, T2W single shot techniques, which provide higher-spatial-resolution anatomic imaging similar to noncontrast CT images than the Dixon-derived images without increasing the overall acquisition time (see **Figs. 4** and **5**). These additional WB-MR imaging sequences are typically used in clinical WB–FDG-PET/MR imaging studies.

In some cases, additional MR imaging sequences for WB imaging may be valuable, particularly for cancers with the potential for variable or low uptake of the PET tracer used in the study. For example, FDG may have reduced sensitivity for densely sclerotic bone metastases compared with lytic metastases; incorporation of a T1 TSE sequence may increase sensitivity for detecting osseous lesions. Similarly, MR imaging sequences, such as STIR and T2 with fat saturation, have high sensitivity for detection of marrow involvement, which may be useful for malignancies, such as multiple myeloma, that have variable FDG uptake. An example of the utility of T1 TSE sequences in multiple myeloma is shown in **Fig. 6**.

DEDICATED REGIONAL MR IMAGING

In addition to WB PET and WB MR imaging, dedicated regional MR imaging is frequently necessary for assessment of locoregional staging and/or assessment of metastatic disease in oncology patients. The ability to simultaneously obtain both PET data and a diagnostic MR examination represents a major advantage of combined PET and MR imaging.[48] For example, WB PET/MR imaging can be coupled with dynamic postcontrast liver MR imaging using a hepatobiliary agent (eg, gadoxetate disodium) in patients with colorectal cancer, thereby effectively staging for nodal disease and unsuspected distant metastases while also greatly improving sensitivity for hepatic metastatic disease.[49,50] Depending on the site of disease, the dedicated regional MR examination can be tailored to the clinical situation. The addition of MR sequences does present challenges, namely, scan time. As others have pointed out, the time required to complete a PET/MR examination should not greatly exceed that of PET/CT with a goal of 60 minutes or less for image acquisition.[51]

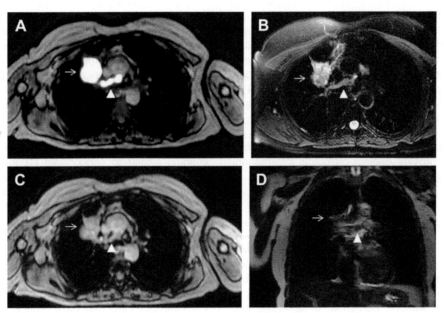

Fig. 5. Use of Dixon sequences for anatomic localization in a patient undergoing initial staging of non–small cell lung cancer. Fused FDG-PET/MR images with coronal opposed-phase (*A*) as well as axial T2-weighted fat saturation (*B*), axial opposed-phase (*C*) and coronal T2 single shot (*D*) MR images are shown. The opposed-phase Dixon images visualize and localize the primary tumor (*white arrowhead*) as well as nodal metastases (*white arrow*). The Dixon sequences are low resolution and provide limited anatomic detail but are adequate in many studies such as this one to localize lesions with increased FDG uptake.[45] However, the Dixon sequences typically are not adequate for primary tumor staging and have limited sensitivity for detection of non–FDG-avid abnormalities. Additional sequences can provide improved soft tissue contrast and higher resolution that are desirable for staging the primary tumor as seen with the T2 FS and single shot images.

The logistics and economics of patient throughput are one consideration; but patient intolerance of prolonged MR studies can severely hinder image quality because of motion artifact, breath-holding difficulties, and overall patient comfort. Hence, modification of existing stand-alone MR protocols must be undertaken in order to limit the total number and length of sequences.

Simplified protocols for liver, pelvic, thoracic, brain, and neck neoplasms have been offered previously[34,48]; but no standardized protocols yet exist. A general approach to accomplish this task, first and foremost, includes removal of sequences that are not essential to answering the clinical question. Additionally, MR techniques, such as a single 3D isotropic acquisition in lieu of multi-planar acquisitions, offer time-savings while maintaining acceptable image resolution on reformatted images. For example, in the evaluation of pelvic malignancy, acquisitions can be reconstructed in orthogonal planes when acquired isotropically as shown in **Fig. 7**. This technique obviates high-resolution imaging in each plane separately but is only effective in regions without substantial motion (eg, head, neck, and pelvis).[34] For clinical PET/MR imaging examinations limited

to one region without a WB component, such as brain and cardiac studies, there is typically less concern about decreasing the total examination time. If a diagnostic MR imaging is performed, the PET image acquisition can be performed during the MR imaging protocol. An example of amyloid-PET/MR imaging is show in **Fig. 8**.

PET PROTOCOL

There are fewer options for PET acquisition compared with the wide variety of MR imaging protocols and sequences, but there are still several important considerations regarding the PET protocol in PET/MR imaging studies. The PET protocol will depend to some extent on the PET tracer used and the clinical application. A list of FDA-approved tracers is presented in **Table 1**. Of note, the recently FDA-approved tracers [^{18}F]fluciclovine for recurrent prostate cancer and [^{68}Ga]DOTATATE for neuroendocrine tumors are particularly well suited for PET/MR imaging. The prostate bed and pelvic lymph nodes are common locations for recurrent prostate cancer, and the liver is a common site of metastases from neuroendocrine tumors. Both of these

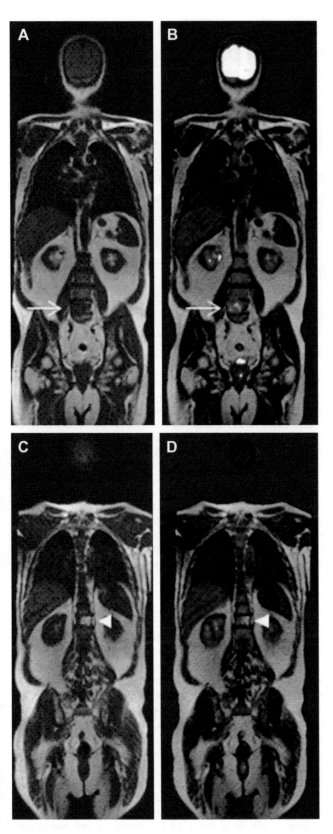

Fig. 6. FDG-PET/MR imaging in a patient with multiple myeloma. Selected coronal T1 TSE images are show in panels (*A*) and (*C*) with corresponding fusion images shown in panels (*B*) and (*D*). An active lesion is seen in a lumbar vertebral body (*white arrow*) with low signal intensity on the T1 TSE MR image (*A*) and increased FDG uptake on the fusion image (*B*). A lesion treated with radiation is seen in a lower thoracic vertebral body (*white arrowhead*) with increased signal intensity on the T1 TSE image (*C*) and decreased FDG uptake (*D*) compared with the rest of the spine because of the replacement of the treated myeloma lesion by fat.

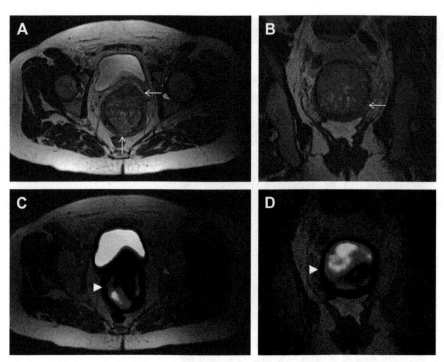

Fig. 7. Near-isotropic high-resolution T2-weighted MR images from a patient undergoing initial staging for cervical cancer. An axial MR image of the pelvis is shown in panel (*A*), and a coronal reformat with minimal loss of resolution is shown in panel (*B*). Corresponding fused FDG-PET/MR images are shown in panels (*C*) and (*D*). The large cervical cancer has markedly increased FDG uptake and is denoted with a white arrowhead. Areas of parametrial invasion are seen as disruption of the hypointense fibrous cervical capsule with lobulated FDG-avid soft tissue with intermediate signal intensity (*white arrows*). The use of near-isotropic sequences in the head, neck, and pelvis provides high-resolution images suitable for multiplanar reformatting and can replace the need for multiple MR imaging acquisitions in different planes for some applications, reducing the overall image acquisition time.

anatomic locations are typically better imaged with MR imaging than with CT. For all PET/MR imaging studies, the duration of PET acquisition per bed position is an important consideration. Typically, a minimum of approximately 2 minutes per position is required for WB FDG-PET studies. However, if the duration of the MR acquisition per bed position is longer than required for adequate counting statistics for PET, the duration of PET acquisition can be extended to reduce image noise or alternatively use a reduced dose of radiopharmaceutical.

For oncologic PET/MR imaging studies with both WB and regional components, the WB acquisition is typically performed first, although some groups perform regional PET/MR imaging first. The primary rationale for performing the WB study first is that patients have been injected with the PET radiopharmaceutical and are committed to the resulting radiation exposure. If the PET/MR imaging study has to be terminated early (eg, technical failure or patient cannot continue), the regional MR imaging can be performed in a separate session without the need to reinject the radiopharmaceutical. When WB followed by regional PET/MR imaging is performed, it is often helpful to perform a second PET acquisition during the regional MR imaging examination, which will facilitate fusion with the regional MR images. Alternatively, if the regional portion of the study is performed first, some or all of the PET tracer uptake time can occur during the regional MR imaging, which will reduce the total time the patients spend in the PET center.

For PET/MR imaging studies involving only one region, such as a neuroimaging or a cardiac study, there is the potential to substantially extend the PET acquisition time and thereby reduce the administered dosage. There is also the possibility of acquiring dynamic and/or multiple time point PET data without extending the overall examination length, which has clear advantages for research PET studies. There is potential diagnostic value for dynamic PET in cardiac perfusion imaging and for neuroimaging, but dynamic and multiple time point PET techniques are not widely used for clinical applications.

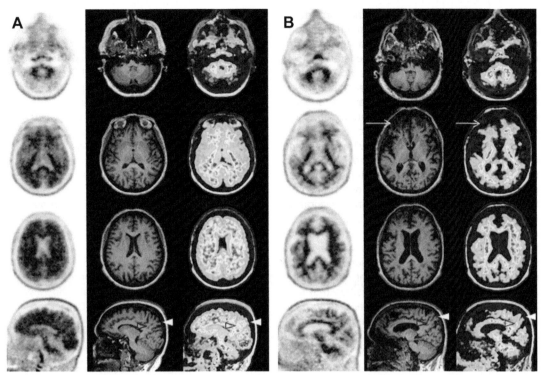

Fig. 8. Amyloid-PET/MR imaging performed with [^{18}F]florbetapir. Representative PET only, fast gradient echo 3D MR images, and fused images in the axial and sagittal plane are shown. (*A*) Positive amyloid PET scan with loss of gray-white differentiation in the cerebral cortex due to abnormally increased amyloid burden. (*B*) Negative amyloid PET scan with maintained gray-white differentiation throughout the cerebral cortex. Although correlation with CT or MR imaging is not required for interpretation of clinical amyloid-PET studies, there are several potential benefits. First, MR imaging provides an excellent depiction of gray and white matter, which can assist with accurately localizing PET tracer accumulation in white versus gray matter. The posterior cingulate (*open red arrowhead*) and precuneus (*solid white arrowhead*) are among the first sites of amyloid deposition, and the sagittal PET/MR imaging fusion image can increase confidence as to whether there is increased amyloid in these regions as in case (*A*). Second, structural abnormalities are readily detect with MR imaging as in the negative case where chronic encephalomalacia is seen in the right frontal lobe (*yellow arrow*). In this case, the loss of gray-white differentiation is due to encephalomalacia rather than increased cortical amyloid. Third, high-resolution 3D MR imaging acquisitions can be used for brain segmentation and measurement of regional brain volumes for defining regions of interest for quantitative PET measurements and for assessing for typical atrophy patterns seen in Alzheimer disease and other neurodegenerative diseases.

ARTIFACTS AND PITFALLS

Many of the artifacts and pitfalls that can occur with PET/CT, such as misregistration, scatter correction errors, and patient motion, can also occur with PET/MR imaging. However, PET/MR imaging has some unique artifacts and potential pitfalls that must be considered. Although PET/CT and MR imaging are affected by metal and attenuation artifacts, the common artifacts observed with PET/MR imaging differ from those seen with PET/CT.[52] Dephasing due to metal or other sources of inhomogeneity in the magnetic field can interfere with the MRAC map, which leads to areas of loss of PET signal. In contrast, CTAC errors with metal and other high-attenuation materials lead to overcorrection of

the PET AC data with resulting artifactually increased SUV measurements. Common sources of these types of errors include dental amalgam, joint arthroplasties, and orthopedic fixation devices. Another type of error that can occur with MRAC is incorrect tissue segmentation that leads to inaccurate AC of the PET data in the affected area. The MRAC map should be reviewed to detect these types of AC errors when reading PET/MRI imaging. For both PET/CT and PET/MR imaging, review of the NAC images is useful when these types of artifacts are present.

A limited 50-cm MR FOV often truncates the arms and in turn generates an incomplete AC map for the 70-cm PET FOV. Inaccurate AC maps generated from truncation can severely affect PET image quality. This truncation artifact can be overcome by using maximum likelihood reconstruction of attenuation and activity techniques that use PET data to generate MRAC maps of regions outside of the MR imaging FOV.[53] There is some suggestion that time-of-flight PET/MR imaging systems have potential to improve MRAC, although this potential has not yet been fully realized in clinical practice.[53,54]

Simultaneous acquisition of PET/MR imaging data can reduce misregistration of the 2 data sets; but in PET/MR imaging, protocols have the potential to have motion errors not present in typical PET/CT studies. Because of the length of PET/MR imaging studies with both WB and regional components, there is greater potential for patient motion over the longer course of the study. A separate PET acquisition during the regional MR imaging component will not be affected by patient changes in position that may have occurred since the WB PET acquisition and are often easier to fuse with the regional MR images. Because many regional MR imaging examinations include multiple breath holds, the regional PET should be acquired before beginning the breath-hold component or, alternatively, correction for respiratory motion must be performed.

SUMMARY

Clinical PET/MR imaging is currently being used as part of routine standard of care around the world. In addition to WB PET and WB MR imaging, dedicated regional MR imaging is frequently necessary for assessment of locoregional staging and/or assessment of metastatic disease in oncology patients. The PET and the MR imaging protocols used for a particular patient depend on the PET tracer used and the clinical question. Overall, careful workflow planning, technologists fluent in the technical aspects of both modalities, WB MR imaging protocols tailored to the clinical question, the overall length of the PET/MR imaging examination, and good communication between the interpreting physicians are all key factors to successful WB PET/MR imaging. PET/MR imaging continues to evolve in terms of data supporting specific indications, and the reimbursement landscape for medical imaging continues to change. Therefore, there is potential for relatively rapid change that may affect the utilization and reimbursement of PET/MR imaging in the near future.

REFERENCES

1. Jadvar H, Subramaniam RM, Berman CG, et al. American College of Radiology and Society of Nuclear Medicine and Molecular Imaging Joint Credentialing Statement for PET/MR Imaging: brain. J Nucl Med 2015;56(4):642–5.
2. Expert Panel on MRS, Kanal E, Barkovich AJ, et al. ACR guidance document on MR safe practices: 2013. J Magn Reson Imaging 2013;37(3):501–30.
3. Ipek EG, Nazarian S. Safety of implanted cardiac devices in an MRI environment. Curr Cardiol Rep 2015;17(7):605.
4. Nordbeck P, Ertl G, Ritter O. Magnetic resonance imaging safety in pacemaker and implantable cardioverter defibrillator patients: how far have we come? Eur Heart J 2015;36(24):1505–11.
5. Camacho JC, Moreno CC, Shah AD, et al. Safety and quality of 1.5-T MRI in patients with conventional and MRI-conditional cardiac implantable electronic devices after implementation of a standardized protocol. AJR Am J Roentgenol 2016;207(3):599–604.
6. Media ACoDaC. ACR manual on contrast media version 10.2. 2016. Available at: http://www.acr.org/~/media/ACR/Documents/PDF/QualitySafety/Resources/Contrast%20Manual/2016_Contrast_Media.pdf. Accessed February 16, 2017.
7. Parikh N, Friedman KP, Shah SN, et al. Practical guide for implementing hybrid PET/MR clinical service: lessons learned from our experience. Abdom Imaging 2015;40(6):1366–73.
8. Ponisio MR, McConathy J, Laforest R, et al. Evaluation of diagnostic performance of whole-body simultaneous PET/MRI in pediatric lymphoma. Pediatr Radiol 2016;46(9):1258–68.
9. Schafer JF, Gatidis S, Schmidt H, et al. Simultaneous whole-body PET/MR imaging in comparison to PET/CT in pediatric oncology: initial results. Radiology 2014;273(1):220–31.
10. Sher AC, Seghers V, Paldino MJ, et al. Assessment of sequential PET/MRI in comparison with PET/CT of pediatric lymphoma: a prospective study. AJR Am J Roentgenol 2016;206(3):623–31.
11. Gatidis S, Schmidt H, Gucke B, et al. Comprehensive oncologic imaging in infants and preschool children with substantially reduced radiation exposure using combined simultaneous (1)(8)F-fluorodeoxyglucose positron emission tomography/magnetic resonance imaging: a direct comparison to (1)(8)F-fluorodeoxyglucose positron emission tomography/computed tomography. Invest Radiol 2016;51(1):7–14.
12. Brix G, Lechel U, Glatting G, et al. Radiation exposure of patients undergoing whole-body dual-modality 18F-FDG PET/CT examinations. J Nucl Med 2005;46(4):608–13.
13. Zeimpekis KG, Barbosa F, Hullner M, et al. Clinical evaluation of PET image quality as a function of acquisition time in a new TOF-PET/MRI compared to TOF-PET/CT–initial results. Mol Imaging Biol 2015;17(5):735–44.

14. Hartung-Knemeyer V, Beiderwellen KJ, Buchbender C, et al. Optimizing positron emission tomography image acquisition protocols in integrated positron emission tomography/magnetic resonance imaging. Invest Radiol 2013;48(5):290–4.

15. Acuff SN, Osborne D. Clinical workflow considerations for implementation of continuous-bed-motion PET/CT. J Nucl Med Technol 2016;44(2):55–8.

16. Sotoudeh H, Sharma A, Fowler KJ, et al. Clinical application of PET/MRI in oncology. J Magn Reson Imaging 2016;44(2):265–76.

17. Hope TA, Verdin EF, Bergsland EK, et al. Correcting for respiratory motion in liver PET/MRI: preliminary evaluation of the utility of bellows and navigated hepatobiliary phase imaging. EJNMMI Phys 2015; 2(1):21.

18. Cabello J, Ziegler SI. Advances in PET/MR instrumentation and image reconstruction. Br J Radiol 2016;20160363. [Epub ahead of print].

19. Manber R, Thielemans K, Hutton B, et al. Initial evaluation of a practical PET respiratory motion correction method in clinical simultaneous PET/MRI. EJNMMI Phys 2014;1(Suppl 1):A40.

20. Dikaios N, Izquierdo-Garcia D, Graves MJ, et al. MRI-based motion correction of thoracic PET: initial comparison of acquisition protocols and correction strategies suitable for simultaneous PET/MRI systems. Eur Radiol 2012;22(2):439–46.

21. Catana C. Motion correction options in PET/MRI. Semin Nucl Med 2015;45(3):212–23.

22. Samarin A, Burger C, Wollenweber SD, et al. PET/MR imaging of bone lesions–implications for PET quantification from imperfect attenuation correction. Eur J Nucl Med Mol Imaging 2012;39(7):1154–60.

23. Eiber M, Takei T, Souvatzoglou M, et al. Performance of whole-body integrated 18F-FDG PET/MR in comparison to PET/CT for evaluation of malignant bone lesions. J Nucl Med 2014;55(2):191–7.

24. Beiderwellen K, Huebner M, Heusch P, et al. Whole-body [(1)(8)F]FDG PET/MRI vs. PET/CT in the assessment of bone lesions in oncological patients: initial results. Eur Radiol 2014;24(8):2023–30.

25. Fraum TJ, Fowler KJ, McConathy J. Conspicuity of FDG-avid osseous lesions on PET/MRI versus PET/CT: a quantitative and visual analysis. Nucl Med Mol Imaging 2016;50(3):228–39.

26. Bruegel M, Gaa J, Woertler K, et al. MRI of the lung: value of different turbo spin-echo, single-shot turbo spin-echo, and 3D gradient-echo pulse sequences for the detection of pulmonary metastases. J Magn Reson Imaging 2007;25(1):73–81.

27. Yi CA, Jeon TY, Lee KS, et al. 3-T MRI: usefulness for evaluating primary lung cancer and small nodules in lobes not containing primary tumors. AJR Am J Roentgenol 2007;189(2):386–92.

28. Biederer J, Schoene A, Freitag S, et al. Simulated pulmonary nodules implanted in a dedicated porcine chest phantom: sensitivity of MR imaging for detection. Radiology 2003;227(2):475–83.

29. Chandarana H, Heacock L, Rakheja R, et al. Pulmonary nodules in patients with primary malignancy: comparison of hybrid PET/MR and PET/CT imaging. Radiology 2013;268(3):874–81.

30. Burris NS, Johnson KM, Larson PE, et al. Detection of small pulmonary nodules with ultrashort echo time sequences in oncology patients by using a PET/MR system. Radiology 2016;278(1):239–46.

31. Koyama H, Ohno Y, Seki S, et al. Magnetic resonance imaging for lung cancer. J Thorac Imaging 2013;28(3):138–50.

32. Kwee TC, Takahara T, Ochiai R, et al. Complementary roles of whole-body diffusion-weighted MRI and 18F-FDG PET: the state of the art and potential applications. J Nucl Med 2010;51(10): 1549–58.

33. Ohno Y, Koyama H, Yoshikawa T, et al. Lung cancer assessment using MR imaging: an update. Magn Reson Imaging Clin N Am 2015;23(2):231–44.

34. Fowler KJ, McConathy J, Narra VR. Whole-body simultaneous positron emission tomography (PET)-MR: optimization and adaptation of MRI sequences. J Magn Reson Imaging 2014;39(2):259–68.

35. Quick HH, von Gall C, Zeilinger M, et al. Integrated whole-body PET/MR hybrid imaging: clinical experience. Invest Radiol 2013;48(5):280–9.

36. Xin J, Ma Q, Guo Q, et al. PET/MRI with diagnostic MR sequences vs PET/CT in the detection of abdominal and pelvic cancer. Eur J Radiol 2016; 85(4):751–9.

37. Beyer T, Lassen ML, Boellaard R, et al. Investigating the state-of-the-art in whole-body MR-based attenuation correction: an intra-individual, inter-system, inventory study on three clinical PET/MR systems. MAGMA 2016;29(1):75–87.

38. Dimopoulos MA, Hillengass J, Usmani S, et al. Role of magnetic resonance imaging in the management of patients with multiple myeloma: a consensus statement. J Clin Oncol 2015;33(6):657–64.

39. Lin C, Luciani A, Itti E, et al. Whole-body diffusion magnetic resonance imaging in the assessment of lymphoma. Cancer Imaging 2012;12:403–8.

40. Olsen JR, Esthappan J, DeWees T, et al. Tumor volume and subvolume concordance between FDG-PET/CT and diffusion-weighted MRI for squamous cell carcinoma of the cervix. J Magn Reson Imaging 2013;37(2):431–4.

41. Ho KC, Lin G, Wang JJ, et al. Correlation of apparent diffusion coefficients measured by 3T diffusion-weighted MRI and SUV from FDG PET/CT in primary cervical cancer. Eur J Nucl Med Mol Imaging 2009; 36(2):200–8.

42. Ohno Y, Koyama H, Onishi Y, et al. Non-small cell lung cancer: whole-body MR examination for M-stage assessment–utility for whole-body

diffusion-weighted imaging compared with integrated FDG PET/CT. Radiology 2008;248(2):643–54.

43. Grueneisen J, Schaarschmidt BM, Beiderwellen K, et al. Diagnostic value of diffusion-weighted imaging in simultaneous 18F-FDG PET/MR imaging for whole-body staging of women with pelvic malignancies. J Nucl Med 2014;55(12):1930–5.

44. Padhani AR, Koh DM, Collins DJ. Whole-body diffusion-weighted MR imaging in cancer: current status and research directions. Radiology 2011; 261(3):700–18.

45. Drzezga A, Souvatzoglou M, Eiber M, et al. First clinical experience with integrated whole-body PET/MR: comparison to PET/CT in patients with oncologic diagnoses. J Nucl Med 2012;53(6): 845–55.

46. Press OW, Li H, Schoder H, et al. US intergroup trial of response-adapted therapy for stage III to IV Hodgkin lymphoma using early interim fluorodeoxyglucose-positron emission tomography imaging: Southwest Oncology Group S0816. J Clin Oncol 2016;34(17):2020–7.

47. Swinnen LJ, Li H, Quon A, et al. Response-adapted therapy for aggressive non-Hodgkin's lymphomas based on early [18F] FDG-PET scanning: ECOG-ACRIN Cancer Research Group study (E3404). Br J Haematol 2015;170(1):56–65.

48. Martinez-Moller A, Eiber M, Nekolla SG, et al. Workflow and scan protocol considerations for integrated whole-body PET/MRI in oncology. J Nucl Med 2012; 53(9):1415–26.

49. Lee KH, Lee JM, Park JH, et al. MR imaging in patients with suspected liver metastases: value of liver-specific contrast agent gadoxetic acid. Korean J Radiol 2013;14(6):894–904.

50. Zech CJ, Herrmann KA, Reiser MF, et al. MR imaging in patients with suspected liver metastases: value of liver-specific contrast agent Gd-EOB-DTPA. Magn Reson Med Sci 2007;6(1):43–52.

51. Fraum TJ, Fowler KJ, McConathy J. PET/MRI: emerging clinical applications in oncology. Acad Radiol 2016;23(2):220–36.

52. Attenberger U, Catana C, Chandarana H, et al. Whole-body FDG PET-MR oncologic imaging: pitfalls in clinical interpretation related to inaccurate MR-based attenuation correction. Abdom Imaging 2015;40(6):1374–86.

53. Boellaard R, Hofman MB, Hoekstra OS, et al. Accurate PET/MR quantification using time of flight MLAA image reconstruction. Mol Imaging Biol 2014;16(4):469–77.

54. Minamimoto R, Levin C, Jamali M, et al. Improvements in PET image quality in time of flight (TOF) simultaneous PET/MRI. Mol Imaging Biol 2016; 18(5):776–81.

Diagnostic Imaging and Newer Modalities for Thoracic Diseases

PET/Computed Tomographic Imaging and Endobronchial Ultrasound for Staging and Its Implication for Lung Cancer

 CrossMark

Sarah J. Counts, DO[a],*, Anthony W. Kim, MD[b]

KEYWORDS

- Chest radiograph • Computed tomography • PET • MRI • Endobronchial ultrasound
- Esophageal ultrasound • Navigational bronchoscopy

KEY POINTS

- Computed tomographic (CT) scanning is the test of choice to identify nodules (ie, low-dose CT scanning) and then to further delineate the abnormality (high-resolution CT scanning).
- Integrated PET/CT imaging is superior to either CT scan or PET imaging by itself in accurately characterizing lung cancers.
- Endobronchial ultrasound and esophageal ultrasound must be used in a strategically advantageous manner relying on their individual strengths to maximize their efficacy in the diagnosis and staging of lung cancer.

INTRODUCTION

Tailoring the optimal diagnostic approach for lung cancer requires that a defined goal be based on the results of any study that is planned. Modalities to detect and characterize lung cancer generally can be divided into those that are invasive versus those that are noninvasive. Aside from the standard chest radiograph (CXR), the noninvasive imaging techniques include computed tomography (CT), PET, and MRI. The invasive imaging modalities include endobronchial ultrasound (EBUS), esophageal ultrasound (EUS), and electromagnetic navigational bronchoscopy (ENB).

NONINVASIVE MODALITIES
Computed Tomographic Scans

- CT scanning is the test of choice to identify nodules (ie, low-dose CT [LDCT] scanning) and then to further delineate the abnormality (ie, high-resolution CT scanning)

The National Lung Screening Trial (NLST) was the landmark prospective randomized, controlled study that revealed a significant decrease in lung cancer–related mortality of 20% when LDCT scans were used (6.8%) compared with CXR alone (26.7%) in the 53,454 participants who were

This article originally appeared in *Surgical Clinics of North America*, Volume 97, Issue 4, August 2017.
The authors have nothing to disclose.
[a] Cardiothoracic Surgery, Yale-New Haven Hospital, Yale School of Medicine, 330 Cedar Street, BB 205, New Haven, CT 06520, USA; [b] Division of Thoracic Surgery, Department of Surgery, Keck School of Medicine, University of Southern California, 1510 San Pablo Street, Suite 514, Los Angeles, CA 90033, USA
* Corresponding author.
E-mail address: sarah.counts@yale.edu

https://doi.org/10.1016/j.cpet.2017.09.003

considered to be at "high risk." High risk was defined in this study as those patients who were current smokers or who were former smokers with a total of 30+ pack-years, aged 55 to 74 years old, as long as they had quit within the past 15 years[1] (**Box 1**). The results of this trial as well as others studies evaluating CXRs for lung cancer screening have led to guidelines recommending its avoidance as a lone screening test for lung cancer because it may miss detecting 4 times as many lung cancers compared with with scans.[2–4] Before the NLST, the International Early Lung Cancer

---

Box 1
Key elements of annual lung screening guidelines endorsed by United States Preventative Services Task Force with further modifications endorsed by the other organizations (endorsing organizations in parentheses)

Inclusion Criteria

Age

   55 to 80 years

   55 to 79 years (AATS)

   55 to 74 years (ACCP, ACS, ASCO, NLST, NCCN)

Tobacco History (ACCP, ACS, ASCO, NLST, NCCN)

   Former smoker with a 30+ pack-year smoking

   Former smoker quit within the past 15 years

   Current smoker

Additional (NCCN, AATS)

   Age 50+ years *and* tobacco history of $\geq$20+ pack-year with at least one additional lung cancer risk factor:

- Major exposure to arsenic, beryllium, oadmium, chromium, nickel, asbestos, coal smoke, soot, silica, and diesel fumes
- Other cancers (small cell lung cancer, head cancers, neck cancers, Hodgkin lymphoma)
- Received radiation treatment to chest for other disease
- Family member with lung cancer (ie, parent, sibling, or child)
- History of COPD
- History of pulmonary fibrosis
- Second-hand smoke exposure

Exclusion Criteria

Age

   Less than 55 years

   Greater than 80 years

Tobacco History

   Less than 30 pack-years

   Quit greater than 15 years ago

Comorbidities (ASCO)

   Severe comorbidities precluding potentially curative treatment and/or limit life expectancy (ASCO)

Discontinuation of Screening

Once a person has not smoked for 15 years or develops a health problem that substantially limits life expectancy or the ability or willingness to have curative lung surgery

Abbreviations: AATS, American Association for Thoracic Surgery; ACCCP, American College of Chest Physicians; ACS, American Cancer Society; ASCO, American Society for Clinical Oncology; COPD, chronic obstructive pulmonary disease; NCCN, National Comprehensive Cancer Network.

Action Program (I-ELCAP) first demonstrated improvements in screening for smokers at high risk for lung cancer.[5] The I-ELCAP subsequently showed that CT imaging detected 4 times more lung cancers and 6 times more stage I lesions as compared with CXR alone when used in the context of screening a higher-risk population.[3–5] Cumulatively and particularly with the results of the NLST, the observed reduction in lung cancer–related mortality now serves as the backbone for the lung cancer screening recommendations from many organizations, including the US Preventive Services Task Force.[1,2,6–11]

From a technical standpoint, a lung cancer screening CT scan should involve low-dose helical (spiral) images from the thoracic inlet moving caudally to the inferior edge of the liver, ensuring that the adrenal glands are included. CT images must be viewed with less than or equal to 2.5-mm slice thickness and with reconstruction intervals less than or equal to slice thickness.[12,13] Additional imaging data may be acquired and reconstructed at less than or equal to 1.0-mm slice thickness and reconstruction intervals to allow for better characterization of small lung nodules.[12] Advanced technology in current iteration CT scanners allows for a high-resolution, comprehensive evaluation of the thorax in a single, several-second breath-hold.[14] Respiratory and cardiac motion artifacts are reduced with rapid acquisition, thereby allowing for more accurate lung nodule depiction, especially in areas that are harder to investigate such as in the bases of the lungs or in the lung parenchyma immediately adjacent to the mediastinum. Newer visualization techniques include maximum intensity projection, volume rendering, stereographic display, and computer-aided detection, which allow for enhanced lung

cancer detection and enable the radiologist to better differentiate small lung nodules from other structures.[14] These technologies have also allowed for multiplanar reconstructions, which can then be used to generate 3-dimensional depictions of vascular and bronchial anatomy for potential future operative planning.

Computed tomographic scans in assessing pulmonary nodules

Pulmonary nodules are one of the most common findings on thoracic imaging, and therefore, it is imperative to make as accurate of a characterization as possible.[15] The size of a pulmonary nodule has been thought to correlate with the prevalence of malignancy: less than 5 mm, 0% to 1%; 5 to 10 mm, 6% to 28%; 10 to 20 mm, 33% to 60%; and greater than 20 mm, 64% to 82%.[16] Although there are variations, the more commonly accepted definition of a pulmonary nodule by CT imaging is a lesion with a diameter less than 30 mm. A pulmonary mass is considered to be a lesion greater than 30 mm.[17]

LDCT identifies small nodules in 10% to 50% of those screened with the vast majority of these being benign.[1–3,18] The wide range seen with nodule detection with CT scanning is not readily explained. Accurate staging for primary lung cancer requires precise demarcation of the tumor margin to assess the primary tumor (T) descriptor, and this delineation is best accomplished with thin-slice high-resolution CT scanning.[13] Therefore, when an LDCT scan identifies a suspicious finding, a dedicated chest high-resolution CT (HRCT) scan should be pursued (**Fig. 1**). LDCT (20–50 mAs) has been shown to be comparable to conventional CT mode (140–300 mAs) in sensitivity and specificity for the detection of pulmonary nodules.[4] There is a significant difference in the

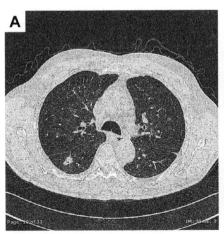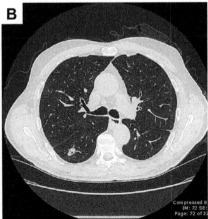

Fig. 1. Differences between low-resolution CT and HRCT scans. (*A*) LDCT scan of the chest with a grainier image and a (*B*) HRCT scan with a more refined image.

radiation in LDCT scanning that ranges from 1.3 to 3.4 mSv, whereas in high-resolution CT imaging, it is 8.5 to 14.0 mSv.[19] In this context, a slice thickness, reconstruction interval of 1.5 to 2.5 mm provides a useful compromise between accurate demarcation of the tumor margin and image noise.[13,20] The noise that is identified typically is an irregular granular pattern in the images, which degrades image information.[21]

Lesions less than 3 mm are extremely difficult to identify on CT imaging because such small abnormalities are difficult to decipher from the lung's normal architecture, especially depending on the location of the presumed nodular finding.[22] The role of nodule location is particularly relevant with small lesions. These lesions are extremely difficult to identify when they are low apparent density or in a central location. Not surprisingly, peripheral lesions are identified more frequently (74%) compared with central (49%) and perihilar lesions (37%), owing to the absence of confounding structures that would be of similar size in the periphery.[22]

Computed tomographic scan in assessing regional lymph nodes

CT scanning has a sensitivity of 47% to 54% and a specificity of 84% to 88% in identifying abnormal hilar and mediastinal lymph nodes with roughly 40% of all nodes thought malignant (as defined by being >1 cm on short-axis diameter) actually being benign and 20% thought benign (as defined by being ≤1 cm on short axis) actually being malignant.[23] Volumetric CT histogram analysis is a relatively new means by which lymph nodes on CT can be evaluated.[24] Flechsig and colleagues[24] demonstrated a significant correlation between lymph node Hounsfield units and benign versus malignant disease with a median CT density being significantly higher for histologically positive lymph nodes (average: 33.2 HU) than for histologically negative lymph nodes (average: 10.1 HU). The incidence of malignancy was 88% above a cutoff value of 20 HU in the 10 fluorine-18 fluorodeoxyglucose (FDG) equivocal lymph nodes, and the incidence of benign findings was 100% in the interval between −20 and +20 HU. Others have noted that there is an increased likelihood of lymph node metastasis if the primary lesion: (1) is solid or spiculated, (2) has a peak enhancement greater than 110 HU, (3) has a net enhancement of greater than 60 to 70 HU on CT scan, (4) is centrally located, or (5) is associated with a pleural effusion.[25,26] Cumulatively, these studies demonstrate promise with respect to the ability of CT scans to distinguish benign from malignant disease, but have not allowed CT scanning to definitively determine if a lymph node harbors metastatic disease.

Integrated PET with Computed Tomography

- Integrated PET/CT imaging is superior to either CT scan or PET imaging by itself in accurately characterizing lung cancers

Integrated PET/CT is the most accurate noninvasive imaging modality for the staging of primary lung cancers.[27,28] Integrated PET/CT refers to when PET is fused with CT scanning and is proven to be a superior imaging modality to either obtained as a sole modality (**Fig. 2**). Current recommendations for PET/CT imaging include obtaining images from the skull base to the thigh with a slice thickness of 2.5 mm to gain the most accurate demarcation of the tumor margin while maximizing the signal-to-noise ratio.[13] PET imaging alone without CT scan fusion is not adequate as a sole modality because it lacks the spatial resolution to accurately and definitely characterize areas of interest.[18,29,30] The paucity of anatomic landmarks on PET imaging is made up for when the images are fused with that of the anatomic cross-sectional data from CT imaging.[31]

The PET component uses an FDG tracer to depict abnormal metabolic uptake with a sensitivity of 79% to 85% and a specificity of 87% to 92% for identifying malignancy.[32] In order to have the PET component have the highest true yield, patients must fast for 4 to 6 hours before the test as well as avoid strenuous activity for 24 to 48 hours before the examination.[13] The FDG tracer is dosed based on the patient's height and weight. Patients with elevated hemoglobin A1c may not be candidates for PET because this can affect the FDG tracer metabolism, with the upper cutoff number varying by institution.

There are areas of the body that have increased uptake of the FDG tracer that are not pathologic, and these must be known so as to not create undue alarm. The most concentrated areas of normal FDG uptake at 1 hour after injection are the brain, heart, and urinary tract. Low-level activity may be seen normally in the thyroid gland, breast, and mediastinal blood pool. Laryngeal uptake can be identified after talking. Physical activity and anxiety can increase uptake within muscle groups in what should be in a symmetric, and if applicable, bilateral fashion.[18] Therefore, a sound grasp of the context in which a PET/CT scan is performed must be understood.

Integrated PET/computed tomography to evaluate the primary lesion

The standardized uptake value (SUV), defined as the activity per milliliter within the region of interest divided by the injected dose in megabecquerels per kilogram of body weight, of a lesion greater

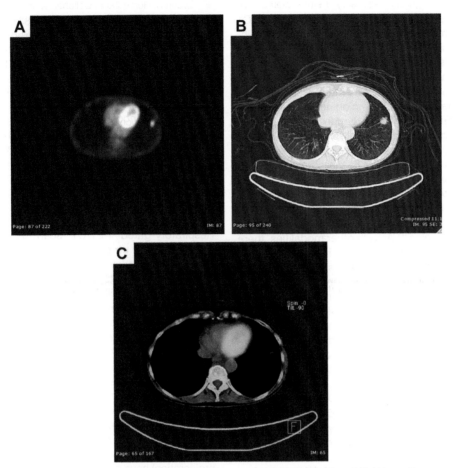

Fig. 2. Differences between a PET scan, CT scan, and integrated PET/CT imaging. (*A*) Attenuation-corrected PET scan, (*B*) CT scan of nodule, (*C*) integrated PET/CT scan of the same nodule.

than 2.5 originally was deemed concerning for malignancy.[30] Since then, the maximum SUV (SUVmax) of greater than 2.5 has been used widely as the cutoff value suggestive of malignancy. This threshold, however, is associated with a wide range of sensitivity (40%–97%) and specificity (60%–96%).[33] This observation may be linked, in part, to false negative results in small nodules (<1 cm) because they may not have the necessary critical mass of metabolically active malignant cells for accurate detection.[34] False negatives occur in small early stage adenocarcinoma, small early squamous cell carcinomas, bronchoalveolar cell carcinoma, and some carcinoid tumors.[35] False positives (nonmalignant lesions with a high SUVmax) also can occur in disease states such as tuberculosis, aspergillomas, rheumatoid nodules, Wegener granulomatosis, and amyloidosis.[35] Cerfolio and colleagues[36] showed that patients with a high SUVmax (≥10) were more likely to have poorly differentiated tumors, more likely to have an advanced stage, and less likely to

undergo complete resection of their disease. Patients with squamous cell carcinoma also were found to have a higher SUVmax (13.2) than those with other types of non–small cell lung cancer (NSCLC 8.9).[36] Despite the potential ominous findings associated with elevated SUVmax, some investigators have shown no difference in overall survival or progression-free survival between high and low SUVmax groups.[37] This finding may be reflective of the heterogeneity in treatment rather than a direct effect of the SUV value, per se. Outside of a quantitative assessment, qualitatively, a nodule or mass with increased uptake of [18]FDG in 3 planes as compared with the background on a PET scan is also concerning for malignancy.[30]

Integrated PET/computed tomographic scans to evaluate lymph node involvement

Similar to the data for primary lung nodules, an SUVmax of 2.5 or greater has been used to differentiate benign from malignant lymph nodes.[38,39]

One prospective, multicenter comparison of CT alone to integrated PET/CT allowed for an 11% increase in accuracy in detecting lymph node metastasis on a per-patient basis.[40] Integrated PET/CT appears to be a better predictor than PET alone for N status.[40] The metabolic characteristics obtained from PET imaging combined with the information regarding lymph node size from CT imaging allows for improved staging accuracy.[41] The risk of mediastinal disease is increased if the SUVmax of the primary lesion is greater than 4.[38]

Integrated PET/CT detects unexpected mediastinal lymph node FDG avidity in 10% of patients originally thought not to have mediastinal disease on other imaging.[41] As with other modalities, there is a risk of false positive findings in mediastinal and hilar lymph nodes. This risk is higher in larger lymph nodes, in those with a higher volume of lymphocytes and macrophages, in reactive lymph nodes, and in those with lymphoid follicular hyperplasia.[40] When the area of concern is small (5–7 mm), the sensitivity of PET drops significantly to only 40% as compared with when investigating larger lymph node stations of concern (8–10 mm) at 78%.[42] Lee and colleagues[43] described lymph node density as an adjunct to FDG avidity in those nodes deemed to have "mild FDG uptake" (SUVmax 2–4), where using density criteria (median HU 25–45) increased the sensitivity (88.3%) and specificity (82.6%) in this subgroup. There are no trials showing a difference in PET/CT imaging between different lung cancer subtypes. A retrospective review by Wang and colleagues[44] found no significant difference in SUVmax on preoperative PET/CT in patients with what was later pathologically proven to be positive lymph node disease between squamous cell carcinoma and other forms of NSCLC.

Integrated PET/computed tomographic scans to delineate metastases

Integrated PET/CT detects unexpected metastases in 10% to 15% of patients with NSCLC.[41] A review of all randomized control trials using PET or PET/CT in the evaluation of patients with lung cancer showed that its greatest benefit was in identifying metastatic disease in patients with a high chance of such involvement.[45] Preoperatively, integrated PET/CT has reduced the total number of thoracotomies including those thoracotomies used for staging in those NSCLC patients presumed to have advanced disease.[30] Integrated PET/CT scans are replacing bone scintigraphy in most cases because it has been shown to be a very sensitive imaging modality to detect osseous disease. One meta-analysis described a higher

sensitivity (92%) and specificity (98%) with integrated PET/CT scanning as compared with bone scintigraphy (sensitivity 86%, specificity 87%) in correctly identifying metastatic disease to bone.[46]

Future advances in integrated PET/computed tomographic imaging

Alternative methods to improve upon current integrated PET/CT imaging are on the horizon. One such approach uses respiratory gating of PET/CT scans, whereby data acquisition corresponds to a specific part of the respiratory cycle phase. This unique approach is different than standard PET/CT techniques, whereby patients are allowed to breathe freely during the examination. Respiratory-gated PET/CT scan use has not been proven to be superior at this time, but has the potential to play a role in the management of patients with early stage disease because it shows slightly improved clinical staging accuracy and higher interobserver agreement between nuclear medicine physicians.[47]

PET imaging using other tracer materials to achieve more sensitive and specific imaging than presently available with [18]FDG is under investigation at this time. A fluorine-18-A-methyltyrosine tracer is currently in clinical trial phases.[48] Other tracers such as 11C-methionine (protein metabolism marker), 11C-choline (a marker of the cell membrane component phosphatidylcholine), and 18F-fluorothymidine (a marker of cell proliferation) have also been studied, but the experience is limited, with no clear clinical advantage identified yet.[49]

INVASIVE EVALUATION

Invasive studies allow the clinician to obtain tissue for both diagnosis and staging. Before using an invasive option for either of these purposes, it is recommended that imaging will have afforded the clinician the knowledge of selecting the target that would provide a diagnosis and the highest possible stage in a safe manner.[50] In certain circumstances, such as in those patients who are suggested to have a peripheral stage IA tumor, invasive preoperative evaluation of mediastinal nodes may not be required.[2,51] However, in general, most abnormal imaging should be confirmed by tissue biopsy using the method that will best ensure accurate staging because evidence shows that more complete staging workups improve patient outcomes.[52–54] In fact, most practice guidelines recommend that patients with a peripheral lesion, defined as being in the outer third of the lung parenchyma, concerning for cancer, require tissue diagnosis before further management can be planned.[55] It is recommended that patients with peripheral pulmonary nodules be considered for a CT-guided transthoracic needle aspiration (TTNA) as an initial diagnostic option.[26,56,57]

Computed Tomographic Imaging to Guide Percutaneous Biopsies

Although CT scans are not used to biopsy lesions, per se, CT still allows for real-time guidance in assessing nodules to allow for percutaneous sampling in the same way an endoscope is used.[58] The indication for biopsy put forth by the I-ELCAP protocol was when a solitary nodule measured 15 mm or more in size, was a solid nodule that had grown on follow-up scans, or was a nonsolid or part-solid nodule that persisted in size and did not resolve on 1- or 3-month follow-up scans.[2,59] More recent guidelines are more stringent and recommend that nodules greater than 8 mm in diameter that have either a pretest probability of malignancy ≥10%, PET avidity, or when a fully informed patient desires a definitive diagnostic procedure, should have a biopsy performed.[2] Additional guidelines for nodules greater than 8 mm also include undergoing a biopsy if there are any data to support a substantial suspicion of lung cancer.[8,10,60]

Transthoracic needle biopsy (TTNB) may provide more information over only the cellular material obtained by TTNA alone because the core needle provides more material by which information regarding cellular architecture and degree of invasiveness can be obtained. The sensitivity of CT-guided TTNB for malignancy ranges from 74% to 97%, and its specificity ranges from 95% to 100%.[58,61–64] A recent review found that CT-guided TTNB was a reliable procedure associated with an 88% to 91% sensitivity for the diagnosis of lung cancer, specifically with the yield being enhanced to 97% when larger core needles (≥18 gauge) were used.[65] If the sample or results of a biopsy are inadequate or inconclusive, respectively, and the suspicion of malignancy remains high, additional biopsy tests should be attempted.[66] Unfortunately, percutaneous procedures also are associated with a significantly higher pneumothorax rate because the needle traverses the pleura and lung.[40,55] These CT-guided transthoracic lung biopsies are associated with an overall incidence of complications that vary greatly (1.7%–45%).[55]

Endoscopically Directed Biopsies

- EBUS and EUS must be used in a strategically advantageous manner relying on their individual strengths to maximize their efficacy in the diagnosis and staging of lung cancer

---

Box 2
Indications for endoscopic biopsies

EBUS

1. Sampling tissue from lung nodule or mass

    R-EBUS if peripheral (outer 1/3)

    L-EBUS if central

    Tissue sampling for biomarker testing (use ROSE if possible)

    Peripheral nodule/mass of any size in a patient with poor surgical candidacy and/or if other techniques are higher risk for that particular patient (ie, CT-guided TTNA in severe bullous chronic obstructive pulmonary disease)

2. Staging patients with lung cancer with mediastinal or hilar lymph node involvement

    Clinical hilar (N1) and/or mediastinal (N2 or N3) disease by CT and/or PET/CT scan

    Central tumor

    Peripheral tumor and >3 cm

3. Confirming pathologic diagnosis of enlarged lymph nodes in suspected or confirmed lymphoproliferative or infectious diseases

4. Evaluating tracheobronchial tree

    Biopsy abnormal tissue

    Assess depth of invasion

5. Sampling tissue from mediastinal nodule or mass

6. Sampling abnormal-appearing tissue concerning for malignant infiltration of the mediastinum

EUS

1. Biopsying left adrenal lesion when concerned for metastasis

2. Biopsying levels 5, 8, and 9 lymph nodes

3. Biopsying of celiac and infradiaphragmatic retroperitoneal lymph nodes

---

The primary advantage of EBUS or EUS over surgical cervical mediastinoscopy is that it can be performed with sedation and rarely requires general anesthesia in skilled hands. Another advantage is that in addition to accessing the mediastinal lymph nodes for sampling, EBUS more so than EUS provides the added advantage of being able to biopsy the hilar lymph nodes and the lung parenchymal lesion itself. EBUS and EUS allow complementary evaluation of almost all mediastinal lymph node levels when combined (**Box 2**).[67]

EUS and EBUS have been shown to be safe techniques with low morbidities and mortalities. Studies of patients undergoing EBUS for peripheral lung nodules have reported an overall low incidence of complication ranging from well under 1%–5%. Specific complications have included pneumothorax (0.8%–2.1%), pulmonary infections (0.5%), and bleeding (1%–5%).[68–72] Deaths due to complications from these procedures are extremely rare (0.04%), with those mortalities occurring in patients with poor preoperative performance status defined by their American Society of Anesthesiologists Physical Status Classification of III or IV.[40]

Advances in on-site tissue sample investigation, referred to as ROSE (ie, Rapid Onsite Evaluation), have also allowed for another advantage with EBUS and EUS in that the biopsies are examined while the patient is undergoing the procedure itself. ROSE of cytology when used with EBUS or EUS sampling has been shown to correlate with 94.8% of lymph nodes having a clear diagnosis on the first pass biopsy as compared with subsequent passes.[73] Therefore, with the addition of ROSE, the need for more than 3 biopsy passes may be unnecessary. The true benefit of ROSE is that the sampled tissue is evaluated in real time

to reduce the rate of nondiagnostic sampling. Furthermore, ROSE has been shown to correlate very well with final pathology and may guide the proceduralist in the order and way the tissues are sampled.[74] If no onsite assessment is available, it is recommended that the needles be changed between sampling of N3, N2, and N1 nodes rather than simply flushing the needles in between sampling of different nodal stations to avoid cross-contamination.[32]

Endobronchial Ultrasound

EBUS was introduced in 1990 and has the advantage of being able to obtain sufficient tissue samples for histologic diagnosis, including immunohistochemistry, which is important in many diseases.[74] Masses adjacent to the airway, intrapulmonary nodules, and mediastinal tumors of unknown cause often times require advanced pathologic diagnosis for definitive diagnosis, and EBUS is able to accomplish this.[40,74]

EBUS uses a radial (R-EBUS) or linear (L-EBUS) probe with a bronchoscope and uses frequencies between 5 and 10 MHz with a penetration at 5 MHz to about 6 to 8 cm (**Fig. 3**).[40,74] The current EBUS iteration includes a dedicated biopsy needle

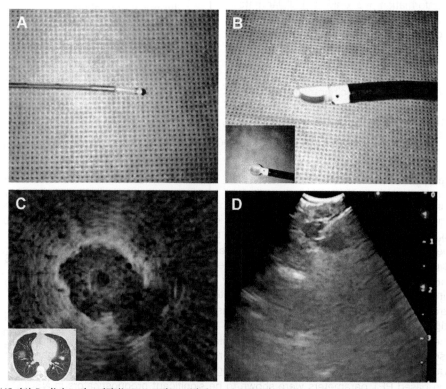

Fig. 3. EBUS. (*A*) Radial probe, (*B*) linear probe with inset image showing balloon expansion, (*C*) ultrasound image of pathologic pulmonary nodule using radial probe with inset showing lesion on CT scan, (*D*) ultrasound image showing needle within a pathologic lymph node using linear probe.

(typically 22 gauge) allowing EBUS-TBNA of levels 2R, 2L, 4R, 4L, 7, 10R, 10L, 11R, and 11L.[40,67,74,75] L-EBUS facilitates TBNA of mediastinal lymph nodes, hilar lymph nodes, intrapulmonary lymph nodes, and central lesions under real-time ultrasound guidance.[76,77] The L-EBUS probe typically is larger than a standard flexible bronchoscope and requires oral intubation.[78] R-EBUS allows for evaluation of central airways and their wall structure (ie, defining airway invasion), hilar lymph nodes, mediastinal lymph nodes, intrapulmonary lymph nodes, and peripheral lung lesions.[33,76,77] The more peripheral intrapulmonary lymph node levels 12 to 14 are also accessible if a miniature R-EBUS probe is used.[67] Small R-EBUS probes (miniprobes) allow for the biopsy of peripheral nodules independent of lesion size with sensitivities ranging from 61% to 80%.[26,77] The further development of even smaller probes with guiding catheters and more advanced miniprobes will solve the navigation issue to move farther into the periphery.[77]

The prevalence of positive mediastinal lymph node disease following a negative EBUS-TBNA is reported to be low at 4.9%.[79] On the other hand, one retrospective study using EBUS sampling for negative CT and PET imaging (ie, unsuspected N2 disease) found that there was an incidence of malignancy in 17.6% of the EBUS samples obtained.[80] Generally, EBUS-TBNA is useful in biopsying centrally located, paratracheal and peribronchial tumors with a diagnostic sensitivity of 82% to 94%.[78]

There are no consistent characteristics on EBUS to predict malignancy. One study suggested that a round or oval shape was correlated with malignancy[73]; however, this has not been universally accepted criteria. Consequently, no particular ultrasound shape characteristic should deter the proceduralist from proceeding with a biopsy. Nevertheless, 3 variables have been correlated strongly with false negative EBUS outcomes: (1) central location of the lung tumor, (2) nodal enlargement on CT, and (3) FDG-avidity for mediastinal lymph nodes on PET imaging.[81]

Endoscopic Ultrasound

EUS-guided biopsy gives the proceduralist the ability to sample lymph nodes that are not accessible via an EBUS approach (levels 5, 8, and 9 lymph nodes and the infradiaphragmatic and retroperitoneal lymph nodes).[67] EUS-guided fine-needle aspiration (FNA) uses a curved linear array ultrasound transducer, which allows for real-time ultrasound-guided needle sampling of the lymph node stations accessible from the esophagus as

well as lung and pleural lesions.[82,83] The location of the esophagus, which is posterior and to the left of the trachea, makes right-sided visualization and sampling more of a challenge even when the lymph nodes are grossly enlarged.[67] The lymph nodes that can be sampled include some of the paratracheal lymph nodes (levels 2R 2L, 4R, and 4L), although anatomic constraints make it challenging to reliably access these levels especially anterior to and to the right of the trachea. Not surprisingly, EUS is associated with an incidence of false negative biopsies in these areas of 19%.[67,82] EUS is better suited for reaching the lymph nodes in the subcarinal (level 7), aortopulmonary window (level 5), periesophageal (level 8), and inferior pulmonary ligament (level 9) stations as well as the infradiaphragmatic retroperitoneal lymph nodes close to the aorta and celiac trunk.[52,67,75,82] EUS-FNA can use a transgastric approach to biopsy abnormalities of the left adrenal glan.[83,84] It is noted that EUS is inferior to transcutaneous ultrasound in the evaluation of the right adrenal gland due to the esophagus's left-sided location.[67]

EUS-guided FNA has been reported to decrease the need for surgical mediastinoscopy by 68% when used as the initial staging tool.[41,83,85] EUS-guided FNA has a sensitivity of 84% to 92.5%, specificity of 89% to 100%, and positive predictive value of 79% to 100% in confirming suspicious mediastinal lymph nodes for malignancy that are detected by FDG-PET in patients with suspected or proven NSCLC.[86] In patients with negative lymph nodes on CT scan (ie, <1 cm), EUS has been shown to identify malignant mediastinal involvement in 25% of those patients as well as identify invasion or left adrenal involvement in 18.75%.[87] Surgical mediastinoscopy continues to have an important role in working up patients with concern for mediastinal lymph node involvement when EBUS/EUS sampling is negative.[2]

Endobronchial Ultrasound Combined with Esophageal Ultrasound

Accurate staging of the disease may be enhanced through combining the EBUS and EUS (EBUS + EUS) techniques. This approach is supported by the results of the Assessment of Surgical Staging versus Endobronchial and Endoscopic Ultrasound in Lung Cancer prospective randomized trial. This study showed a sensitivity of 79% for detecting mediastinal lymph node metastasis with immediate surgical staging alone versus 85% for EUS + EBUS only.[88] The same study showed that when EUS + EBUS was negative followed by immediate surgical mediastinoscopy to confirm this finding, the sensitivity was 94%.[88] Ultimately, this approach resulted in fewer thoracotomies. It was determined that 11 patients needed to undergo mediastinoscopy in order to detect one single patient with N2 disease missed by combined EBUS + EUS.[88] These findings may represent a point in the evolution of a possible enhanced role in combined endoscopic modalities that may challenge surgical staging in the future.

Electromagnetic Navigational Bronchoscopy

ENB was approved for use in 2004 and is used to evaluate lesions that are peripherally located beyond the depth that a traditional bronchoscope can reach.[89] This technique uses an electromagnetic array to create an electromagnetic field around the patient with a computer system that then uses a preoperative CT scan to provide the bronchoscopic probe location on a screen in 3 dimensions.[90] It combines conventional and virtual bronchoscopy to enable the guidance of bronchoscopic instruments to target areas within the peripheral lung parenchyma.[91] This system is analogous to a Global Positioning System that is used to guide an automobile's navigation. The navigation system shows a "road map" of the bronchial tree on the display screen that the proceduralist can follow. The diagnostic yield of this technique for biopsying these peripheral lesions varies widely and is reported to range from 55.7% to 94%.[91–93]

Other uses for ENB have also included marking peripheral lesions with dye, placing fiducials for nonpalpable lesions before planned thoracoscopic resections, and placing brachytherapy catheters.[91,92] Relatively small series have demonstrated complete success when using ENB for localizing and resecting lung parenchymal lesions.[92] Although promising, refinements to ENB are needed to fully define the scope of its applicability.

DISCUSSION

In terms of noninvasive studies, although CXRs have been the historical workhorse in evaluating patients with lung cancer, CT scanning has become the diagnostic imaging study that has allowed for the greatest anatomic detail. Integrated PET/CT scanning has now emerged as an important adjunct to imaging for lung cancer because of its sensitivity in detecting metabolic activity that would be suggestive of malignancy. Other modalities and advances in imaging either have been shown to be inferior to these 2 imaging modalities or have yet to supplant these 2

modalities as the mainstays in the workup of patients with lung cancer. Nevertheless, more data regarding the refinements in these modalities surely will hone their utility in the diagnosis and staging of lung cancer. With respect to invasive studies, EBUS and EUS techniques are evolving modalities that are approaching the effectiveness, particularly when used in conjunction, that is rivaling more traditional surgical diagnostic and staging procedures. Furthermore, advances such as ENB have the potential to steer innovation down new exciting avenues.

SUMMARY

In summary, CXR, although useful in detecting some thoracic abnormalities, should not be part of a formal screening or staging protocol exclusively. Rather, LDCT scanning should be used to screen for lung cancer in high-risk patients as defined by national and international guidelines. Once an abnormality is identified by screening LDCT, additional imaging should be performed with HRCT scanning to characterize the abnormality in greater detail. If concern for a malignancy remains, a follow-up PET/CT scan should be used to further delineate the lesion as well as complete noninvasive staging through the assessment of the mediastinum and the identification of, or lack thereof, possible metastatic disease. Mediastinal involvement of disease then can be confirmed by minimally invasive techniques such as EBUS and EUS. In experienced hands, these techniques are approaching an efficacy similar to that of cervical mediastinoscopy in being the definitive invasive staging procedure. EBUS may provide the additional benefit over cervical mediastinoscopy of allowing the clinician to achieve a tissue diagnosis of the pulmonary lesion during the same setting of mediastinal staging.

REFERENCES

1. National Lung Screening Trial Research Trial, Aberle DR, Adams AM, et al. Reduced lung-cancer mortality with low-dose computed tomographic screening. N Engl J Med 2011;365(5): 395–409.
2. Detterbeck FC, Mazzone PJ, Naidich DP, et al. Screening for lung cancer: diagnosis and management of lung cancer, 3rd ed: American College of Chest Physicians evidence-based clinical practice guidelines. Chest 2013;143(5 Suppl):e78S–92S.
3. Henschke CI, McCauley DI, Yankelevitz DF, et al. Early Lung Cancer Action Project: overall design and findings from baseline screening. Lancet 1999;354(9173):99–105.

4. Midthun DE, Jett JR. Screening for lung cancer: the US studies. J Surg Oncol 2013;108(5):275–9.
5. Henschke CI, Yankelevitz DF, Kostis WJ. CT screening for lung cancer. Semin Ultrasound CT MR 2003;24(1):23–32.
6. Rocco G, Allen MS, Altorki NK, et al. Clinical statement on the role of the surgeon and surgical issues relating to computed tomography screening programs for lung cancer. Ann Thorac Surg 2013; 96(1):357–60.
7. Bach PB, Mirkin JN, Oliver TK, et al. Benefits and harms of CT screening for lung cancer: a systematic review. JAMA 2012;307(22):2418–29.
8. Jaklitsch MT, Jacobson FL, Austin JH, et al. The American Association for Thoracic Surgery guidelines for lung cancer screening using low-dose computed tomography scans for lung cancer survivors and other high-risk groups. J Thorac Cardiovasc Surg 2012;144(1):33–8.
9. Wood DE, Eapen GA, Ettinger DS, et al. Lung cancer screening. J Natl Compr Cancer Netw 2012; 10(2):240–65.
10. Wood DE. National Comprehensive Cancer Network (NCCN) clinical practice guidelines for lung cancer screening. Thorac Surg Clin 2015; 25(2):185–97.
11. Moyer VA, Force USPST. Screening for lung cancer: U.S. Preventive Services Task Force recommendation statement. Ann Intern Med 2014;160(5):330–8.
12. Fischbach F, Knollmann F, Griesshaber V, et al. Detection of pulmonary nodules by multislice computed tomography: improved detection rate with reduced slice thickness. Eur Radiol 2003; 13(10):2378–83.
13. Paul NS, Ley S, Metser U. Optimal imaging protocols for lung cancer staging: CT, PET, MR imaging, and the role of imaging. Radiol Clin North Am 2012;50(5):935–49.
14. Lee WK, Lau EW, Chin K, et al. Modern diagnostic and therapeutic interventional radiology in lung cancer. J Thorac Dis 2013;5(Suppl 5): S511–23.
15. Sieren JC, Ohno Y, Koyama H, et al. Recent technological and application developments in computed tomography and magnetic resonance imaging for improved pulmonary nodule detection and lung cancer staging. J Magn Reson Imaging 2010;32(6): 1353–69.
16. Wahidi MM, Govert JA, Goudar RK, et al, American College of Chest Physicians. Evidence for the treatment of patients with pulmonary nodules: when is it lung cancer?: ACCP evidence-based clinical practice guidelines (2nd edition). Chest 2007;132(3 Suppl):94S–107S.
17. Hansell DM, Bankier AA, MacMahon H, et al. Fleischner Society: glossary of terms for thoracic imaging. Radiology 2008;246(3):697–722.
18. Devaraj A, Cook GJ, Hansell DM. PET/CT in non-small cell lung cancer staging-promises and problems. Clin Radiol 2007;62(2):97–108.
19. Ono K, Hiraoka T, Ono A, et al. Low-dose CT scan screening for lung cancer: comparison of images and radiation doses between low-dose CT and follow-up standard diagnostic CT. Springerplus 2013;2:393.
20. Henschke CI, Yankelevitz DF, Smith JP, et al. Screening for lung cancer: the early lung cancer action approach. Lung Cancer 2002;35(2):143–8.
21. Goldman LW. Principles of CT: radiation dose and image quality. J Nucl Med Technol 2007;35(4):213–25 [quiz: 226–8].
22. Naidich DP, Rusinek H, McGuinness G, et al. Variables affecting pulmonary nodule detection with computed tomography: evaluation with three-dimensional computer simulation. J Thorac Imaging 1993;8(4):291–9.
23. Silvestri GA, Gould MK, Margolis ML, et al. Noninvasive staging of non-small cell lung cancer: ACCP evidenced-based clinical practice guidelines (2nd edition). Chest 2007;132(3 Suppl): 178S–201S.
24. Flechsig P, Kratochwil C, Schwartz LH, et al. Quantitative volumetric CT-histogram analysis in N-staging of 18F-FDG-equivocal patients with lung cancer. J Nucl Med 2014;55(4):559–64.
25. Tsim S, O'Dowd CA, Milroy R, et al. Staging of non-small cell lung cancer (NSCLC): a review. Respir Med 2010;104(12):1767–74.
26. Detterbeck FC, Jantz MA, Wallace M, et al. Invasive mediastinal staging of lung cancer: ACCP evidence-based clinical practice guidelines (2nd edition). Chest 2007;132(3 Suppl):202S–20S.
27. Schrevens L, Lorent N, Dooms C, et al. The role of PET scan in diagnosis, staging, and management of non-small cell lung cancer. Oncologist 2004; 9(6):633–43.
28. Toba H, Kondo K, Otsuka H, et al. Diagnosis of the presence of lymph node metastasis and decision of operative indication using fluorodeoxyglucose-positron emission tomography and computed tomography in patients with primary lung cancer. J Med Invest 2010;57(3–4):305–13.
29. Lardinois D, Weder W, Hany TF, et al. Staging of non-small-cell lung cancer with integrated positron-emission tomography and computed tomography. N Engl J Med 2003;348(25):2500–7.
30. Fischer B, Lassen U, Mortensen J, et al. Preoperative staging of lung cancer with combined PET-CT. N Engl J Med 2009;361(1):32–9.
31. von Schulthess GK, Steinert HC, Hany TF. Integrated PET/CT: current applications and future directions. Radiology 2006;238(2):405–22.
32. Fielding DI, Kurimoto N. EBUS-TBNA/staging of lung cancer. Clin Chest Med 2013;34(3):385–94.

33. Mattes MD, Moshchinsky AB, Ahsanuddin S, et al. Ratio of lymph node to primary tumor SUV on PET/CT accurately predicts nodal malignancy in non-small-cell lung cancer. Clin Lung Cancer 2015; 16(6):e253–8.

34. Kitajima K, Doi H, Kanda T, et al. Present and future roles of FDG-PET/CT imaging in the management of lung cancer. Jpn J Radiol 2016;34(6):387–99.

35. Rankin S. PET/CT for staging and monitoring non small cell lung cancer. Cancer Imaging 2008;8 Spec No A:S27–31.

36. Cerfolio RJ, Bryant AS, Ohja B, et al. The maximum standardized uptake values on positron emission tomography of a non-small cell lung cancer predict stage, recurrence, and survival. J Thorac Cardiovasc Surg 2005;130(1):151–9.

37. Kim SJ, Chang S. Limited prognostic value of SUV max measured by F-18 FDG PET/CT in newly diagnosed small cell lung cancer patients. Oncol Res Treat 2015;38(11):577–85.

38. Moloney F, Ryan D, McCarthy L, et al. Increasing the accuracy of 18F-FDG PET/CT interpretation of "mildly positive" mediastinal nodes in the staging of non small cell lung cancer. Eur J Radiol 2014; 83(5):843–7.

39. Hellwig D, Graeter TP, Ukena D, et al. 18F-FDG PET for mediastinal staging of lung cancer: which SUV threshold makes sense? J Nucl Med 2007;48(11): 1761–6.

40. Dietrich CF, Annema JT, Clementsen P, et al. Ultrasound techniques in the evaluation of the mediastinum, part I: endoscopic ultrasound (EUS), endobronchial ultrasound (EBUS) and transcutaneous mediastinal ultrasound (TMUS), introduction into ultrasound techniques. J Thorac Dis 2015;7(9): E311–25.

41. Tournoy KG, Carprieaux M, Deschepper E, et al. Are EUS-FNA and EBUS-TBNA specimens reliable for subtyping non-small cell lung cancer? Lung Cancer 2012;76(1):46–50.

42. Reinhardt MJ, Wiethoelter N, Matthies A, et al. PET recognition of pulmonary metastases on PET/CT imaging: impact of attenuation-corrected and non-attenuation-corrected PET images. Eur J Nucl Med Mol Imaging 2006;33(2):134–9.

43. Lee SM, Goo JM, Park CM, et al. Preoperative staging of non-small cell lung cancer: prospective comparison of PET/MR and PET/CT. Eur Radiol 2016; 26(11):3850–7.

44. Wang Y, Ma S, Dong M, et al. Evaluation of the factors affecting the maximum standardized uptake value of metastatic lymph nodes in different histological types of non-small cell lung cancer on PET-CT. BMC Pulm Med 2015;15:20.

45. Detterbeck FC, Figueroa Almanzar S. Lung cancer staging: the value of PET depends on the clinical setting. J Thorac Dis 2014;6(12):1714–23.

46. Qu X, Huang X, Yan W, et al. A meta-analysis of (1)(8)FDG-PET-CT, (1)(8)FDG-PET, MRI and bone scintigraphy for diagnosis of bone metastases in patients with lung cancer. Eur J Radiol 2012;81(5): 1007–15.

47. Grootjans W, Hermsen R, van der Heijden EH, et al. The impact of respiratory gated positron emission tomography on clinical staging and management of patients with lung cancer. Lung Cancer 2015; 90(2):217–23.

48. Kaira K, Oriuchi N, Otani Y, et al. Fluorine-18-alpha-methyltyrosine positron emission tomography for diagnosis and staging of lung cancer: a clinicopathologic study. Clin Cancer Res 2007;13(21):6369–78.

49. Wynants J, Stroobants S, Dooms C, et al. Staging of lung cancer. Radiol Clin North Am 2007;45(4): 609–25, v.

50. Evison M, Crosbie P, Booton R. Should all lung cancer patients requiring mediastinal staging with EBUS undergo PET-CT first? J Bronchology Interv Pulmonol 2015;22(2):e5–7.

51. Darling GE, Dickie AJ, Malthaner RA, et al. Invasive mediastinal staging of non-small-cell lung cancer: a clinical practice guideline. Curr Oncol 2011;18(6): e304–10.

52. Silvestri GA, Gonzalez AV, Jantz MA, et al. Methods for staging non-small cell lung cancer: diagnosis and management of lung cancer, 3rd ed: American College of Chest Physicians evidence-based clinical practice guidelines. Chest 2013;143(5 Suppl): e211S–250S.

53. Vilmann P, Clementsen PF, Colella S, et al. Combined endobronchial and oesophageal endosonography for the diagnosis and staging of lung cancer. European Society of Gastrointestinal Endoscopy (ESGE) Guideline, in cooperation with the European Respiratory Society (ERS) and the European Society of Thoracic Surgeons (ESTS). Eur Respir J 2015; 46(1):40–60.

54. Novello S, Barlesi F, Califano R, et al. Metastatic non-small-cell lung cancer: ESMO Clinical Practice Guidelines for diagnosis, treatment and follow-up. Ann Oncol 2016;27(Suppl 5):v1–27.

55. Heerink WJ, de Bock GH, de Jonge GJ, et al. Complication rates of CT-guided transthoracic lung biopsy: meta-analysis. Eur Radiol 2016;27(1):138–48.

56. Ost DE, Gould MK. Decision making in patients with pulmonary nodules. Am J Respir Crit Care Med 2012;185(4):363–72.

57. Ettinger D, et al. NCCN Clinical Practice Guidelines in Oncology (NCCN Guidelines), Non-Small Cell Lung Cancer. Version 7.2015. 2015; Version 7.2015: NCCN Clinical Practice Guidelines in Oncology (NCCN Guidelines), Non-Small Cell Lung Cancer. Available at: https://www.tri-kobe.org/nccn/guideline/lung/english/non_small.pdf. Accessed October 31, 2016.

58. Ghaye B, Dondelinger RF. Imaging guided thoracic interventions. Eur Respir J 2001;17(3):507–28.

59. Wagnetz U, Menezes RJ, Boerner S, et al. CT screening for lung cancer: implication of lung biopsy recommendations. AJR Am J Roentgenol 2012; 198(2):351–8.

60. Vansteenkiste J, De Ruysscher D, Eberhardt WE, et al. Early and locally advanced non-small-cell lung cancer (NSCLC): ESMO Clinical Practice Guidelines for diagnosis, treatment and follow-up. Ann Oncol 2013;24(Suppl 6):vi89–98.

61. Larscheid RC, Thorpe PE, Scott WJ. Percutaneous transthoracic needle aspiration biopsy: a comprehensive review of its current role in the diagnosis and treatment of lung tumors. Chest 1998;114(3): 704–9.

62. Toloza EM, Harpole L, Detterbeck F, et al. Invasive staging of non-small cell lung cancer: a review of the current evidence. Chest 2003;123(1 Suppl): 157S–66S.

63. Rivera MP, Mehta AC, Wahidi MM. Establishing the diagnosis of lung cancer: diagnosis and management of lung cancer, 3rd ed: American College of Chest Physicians evidence-based clinical practice guidelines. Chest 2013;143(5 Suppl): e142S–65S.

64. de Margerie-Mellon C, de Bazelaire C, de Kerviler E. Image-guided biopsy in primary lung cancer: why, when and how. Diagn Interv Imaging 2016;97(10): 965–72.

65. Loubeyre P, Copercini M, Dietrich PY. Percutaneous CT-guided multisampling core needle biopsy of thoracic lesions. AJR Am J Roentgenol 2005; 185(5):1294–8.

66. Fontaine-Delaruelle C, Souquet PJ, Gamondes D, et al. Negative predictive value of transthoracic core-needle biopsy: a multicenter study. Chest 2015;148(2):472–80.

67. Jenssen C, Annema JT, Clementsen P, et al. Ultrasound techniques in the evaluation of the mediastinum, part 2: mediastinal lymph node anatomy and diagnostic reach of ultrasound techniques, clinical work up of neoplastic and inflammatory mediastinal lymphadenopathy using ultrasound techniques and how to learn mediastinal endosonography. J Thorac Dis 2015;7(10): E439–58.

68. Hayama M, Izumo T, Matsumoto Y, et al. Complications with endobronchial ultrasound with a guide sheath for the diagnosis of peripheral pulmonary lesions. Respiration 2015;90(2): 129–35.

69. Dong X, Qiu X, Liu Q, et al. Endobronchial ultrasound-guided transbronchial needle aspiration in the mediastinal staging of non-small cell lung cancer: a meta-analysis. Ann Thorac Surg 2013;96(4): 1502–7.

70. Bernasconi M, Casutt A, Koutsokera A, et al. Radial ultrasound-assisted transbronchial biopsy: a new diagnostic approach for non-resolving pulmonary infiltrates in neutropenic hemato-oncological patients. Lung 2016;194(6):917–21.

71. Georgiou HD, Taverner J, Irving LB, et al. Safety and efficacy of radial EBUS for the investigation of peripheral pulmonary lesions in patients with advanced COPD. J Bronchology Interv Pulmonol 2016;23(3): 192–8.

72. Zamora FD, Moughrabieh A, Gibson H, et al. An expectorated "stent": an unexpected complication of EBUS-TBNA. J Bronchology Interv Pulmonol 2016. [Epub ahead of print].

73. Memoli JS, El-Bayoumi E, Pastis NJ, et al. Using endobronchial ultrasound features to predict lymph node metastasis in patients with lung cancer. Chest 2011;140(6):1550–6.

74. Nakajima T, Yasufuku K, Yoshino I. Current status and perspective of EBUS-TBNA. Gen Thorac Cardiovasc Surg 2013;61(7):390–6.

75. Gelberg J, Grondin S, Tremblay A. Mediastinal staging for lung cancer. Can Respir J 2014;21(3): 159–61.

76. Gomez M, Silvestri GA. Endobronchial ultrasound for the diagnosis and staging of lung cancer. Proc Am Thorac Soc 2009;6(2):180–6.

77. Zaric B, Stojsic V, Sarcev T, et al. Advanced bronchoscopic techniques in diagnosis and staging of lung cancer. J Thorac Dis 2013;5(Suppl 4): S359–70.

78. Anantham D, Koh MS, Ernst A. Endobronchial ultrasound. Respir Med 2009;103(10):1406–14.

79. Taverner J, Cheang MY, Antippa P, et al. Negative EBUS-TBNA predicts very low prevalence of mediastinal disease in staging of non-small cell lung cancer. J Bronchology Interv Pulmonol 2016;23(2): 177–80.

80. Shingyoji M, Nakajima T, Yoshino M, et al. Endobronchial ultrasonography for positron emission tomography and computed tomography-negative lymph node staging in non-small cell lung cancer. Ann Thorac Surg 2014;98(5):1762–7.

81. Talebian Yazdi M, Egberts J, Schinkelshoek MS, et al. Endosonography for lung cancer staging: predictors for false-negative outcomes. Lung Cancer 2015;90(3):451–6.

82. Khoo KL, Ho KY. Endoscopic mediastinal staging of lung cancer. Respir Med 2011;105:515–8.

83. Colella S, Vilmann P, Konge L, et al. Endoscopic ultrasound in the diagnosis and staging of lung cancer. Endosc Ultrasound 2014;3(4): 205–12.

84. Eloubeidi MA. Endoscopic ultrasound-guided fine-needle aspiration in the staging and diagnosis of patients with lung cancer. Semin Thorac Cardiovasc Surg 2007;19(3):206–11.

85. Tournoy KG, Ryck FD, Vanwalleghem L, et al. The yield of endoscopic ultrasound in lung cancer staging: does lymph node size matter? J Thorac Oncol 2008;3(3):245–9.

86. Eloubeidi MA, Cerfolio RJ, Chen VK, et al. Endoscopic ultrasound-guided fine needle aspiration of mediastinal lymph node in patients with suspected lung cancer after positron emission tomography and computed tomography scans. Ann Thorac Surg 2005;79(1):263–8.

87. Wallace MB, Ravenel J, Block MI, et al. Endoscopic ultrasound in lung cancer patients with a normal mediastinum on computed tomography. Ann Thorac Surg 2004;77(5):1763–8.

88. Annema JT, van Meerbeeck JP, Rintoul RC, et al. Mediastinoscopy vs endosonography for mediastinal nodal staging of lung cancer: a randomized trial. JAMA 2010;304(20):2245–52.

89. Kalanjeri S, Gildea TR. Electromagnetic navigational bronchoscopy for peripheral pulmonary nodules. Thorac Surg Clin 2016;26(2):203–13.

90. Bauer TL, Berkheim DB. Bronchoscopy: diagnostic and therapeutic for non-small cell lung cancer. Surg Oncol Clin N Am 2016;25(3):481–91.

91. Goud A, Dahagam C, Breen DP, et al. Role of electromagnetic navigational bronchoscopy in pulmonary nodule management. J Thorac Dis 2016; 8(Suppl 6):S501–8.

92. Awais O, Reidy MR, Mehta K, et al. Electromagnetic navigation bronchoscopy-guided dye marking for thoracoscopic resection of pulmonary nodules. Ann Thorac Surg 2016;102:223–9.

93. Gildea TR, Mazzone PJ, Karnak D, et al. Electromagnetic navigation diagnostic bronchoscopy: a prospective study. Am J Respir Crit Care Med 2006;174(9):982–9.